F̶r̶ ̶ ̶ ̶ ̶ ̶ ̶ ̶ ̶ ̶ent

Theory

Enhancement Orthodontics

Theory and Practice

Marc Bernard Ackerman, DMD
Diplomate, American Board of Orthodontics
Clinical Associate Professor
Temple University School of Dentistry
Department of Orthodontics
Philadelphia, Pennsylvania
Private Practice of Orthodontics
Bryn Mawr, Pennsylvania

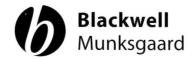
Blackwell
Munksgaard

Editorial Offices:
Blackwell Publishing Professional,
2121 State Avenue, Ames, Iowa 50014-8300, USA
 Tel: +1 515 292 0140
9600 Garsington Road, Oxford OX4 2DQ
 Tel: 01865 776868
Blackwell Publishing Asia Pty Ltd,
550 Swanston Street, Carlton South,
Victoria 3053, Australia
 Tel: +61 (0)3 9347 0300
Blackwell Wissenschafts Verlag, Kurfürstendamm 57, 10707 Berlin, Germany
 Tel: +49 (0)30 32 79 060

First published 2007 by Blackwell Munksgaard, a Blackwell Publishing Company

Library of Congress
Cataloging-in-Publication Data
Ackerman, Marc.
 Enhancement orthodontics : theory and practice / Marc Ackerman.
 – 1st ed.
   p. ; cm.
 Includes bibliographical references.
 ISBN-13: 978-0-8138-2623-3 (alk. paper)
 ISBN-10: 0-8138-2623-3 (alk. paper)
 1. Orthodontics. 2. Dentistry–Aesthetic aspects. I. Title.
 [DNLM: 1. Malocclusion–therapy. 2. Esthetics, Dental. 3. Orthodontics,
Corrective–methods. WU 440 A182e 2007]
 RK521.A 25 2007
 617.6′43–dc22

2006033061

0-8138-2623-3

Set in 10 on 12 pt Sabon
by SNP Best-set Typesetter Ltd., Hong Kong
Printed and bound by C.O.S. Printers Pte Ltd

For further information on
Blackwell Publishing, visit our website:
www.blackwellpublishing.com

To my soulmate, Vanessa,
and
My precious daughter, Olivia Elizabeth

Contents

Foreword

It is fascinating to see the efforts of a third-generation orthodontist examining the history of his specialty and attempting to help his colleagues build on the contributions of the past and create a new future. The author learned much about dentistry sitting at the feet of his grandfather and father and also benefited tremendously from his dental education, where he was exposed to the teachings of Morton Amsterdam, Robert Tisot, and several other legends who comprised the faculty of the University of Pennsylvania School of Dental Medicine at the end of the twentieth century.

At times, the author appears to be an iconoclast as he examines the writings of the fathers of orthodontics, but he has the unique talent of taking important and time-honored valuable information and blending it with more recent data to help clinicians put their treatment plans on a sound biological basis that embraces the technology and evidence of the twenty-first century. The quality of understanding and reviewing the history of a discipline is extremely useful in contributing to the teaching and advances of a subject and thus an important strength of this volume.

One of the critical themes of this book is the belief that there is more to orthodontics than the occlusion of the dentition. A major part of this writing is devoted to the total evaluation of the patient. The author goes to great lengths to detail the examination procedures, not only intraorally but also the extraoral evaluation of the face and particularly the individual's smile. The methodology involved in the clinical examination of dentofacial traits is carefully described in Chapter 3. The reader is given detailed techniques to observe and classify these characteristics, and great attention is devoted to the different aspects of the patient's smile. The collected data relative to the examination of dentofacial tissues and the smile are described with methods useful to the therapist. In the patient evaluation, great emphasis is placed on the patient's wishes as well as his or her needs. Bringing the patient's desires into consideration is of tremendous importance because treatment actually places the individual in the role of co-management with the therapist. This is obvious not only in the area of personal oral hygiene but also with compliance in the long-term maintenance phase. The author also reflects his training by stressing the recognition of periodontal health as well as the use of materials, which play a major role in the maintenance of the case.

The major part of this text is devoted to studying the patient in great detail. The collection of data prepares the therapist to develop a treatment plan, and significant time goes into this phase. Chapter 2, Communication in Orthodontics, is masterfully presented and has great application to all aspects of dental medicine. When one observes the section devoted to the examination and evaluation of the face and the smile, it is clear that this information not only is of great value to the orthodontist but also has great importance in the treatment of the advanced restorative cases considered for periodontal prosthesis and other major oral restorations. One sees the benefit of utilizing these chapters in teaching residents and graduate students in prosthodontics and restorative dentistry. Bringing the patient's wishes into the evaluation procedures should apply to all areas of dental medicine.

The variety of cases discussed in Chapter 6 enables the reader to see the synthesis of information gained in earlier chapters and applied to the patient. The illustrations are quite useful and well done, and the descriptions of the enhancements for each case are of value to the student. It is refreshing to have a new text in this field that is not advocating new appliances or materials in solving the problems of patients. The author is to be praised for bringing this information to the attention of the profession and introducing it in the new and modern orthodontics.

The information provided in this text has been used in the author's clinical practice and has been part of his teaching activities with postdoctoral orthodontic students with great success. Dr. Ackerman's contribution to the literature and his presentations at scientific meetings have been received with enthusiasm and strong interest.

D. Walter Cohen, DDS
Dean-Emeritus, University of Pennsylvania
School of Dental Medicine
Chancellor-Emeritus, Drexel University
College of Medicine

Preface

Enhancement Orthodontics: Theory and Practice represents the encapsulation of a 10-year odyssey in search of clarification as to what defines orthodontic health and orthodontic need. It has been colored by my experiences in orthodontic residency, private practice, research, lecturing, and teaching. Before applying to orthodontic residency in 1997, I posed a single question to my father, a second-generation orthodontist: "Does orthodontics really work?" He irreverently answered, "No, not really." From that point forward, we engaged in an ongoing conversation discussing the nature of orthodontics and the reasons why patients seek our services. After 10 years, I can finally appreciate his markedly cynical answer related to success in clinical practice. The root of frustration has been our inability to reconcile the fact that patients approach orthodontic health, orthodontic need, and orthodontic outcome from an entirely different perspective than orthodontists.

The enhancement orthodontic model presented in this work offers a fresh perspective on the nature of orthodontics and its role in contemporary society. The reader will learn that success in orthodontic treatment is dependent on striking a balance between servicing the needs of the patient and exercising sound professional judgment. In order for the orthodontist to achieve any level of success, they must regard the patient as a co-decision maker. When practiced in this interactive patient-centered model, I am pleased to say that orthodontics does indeed "work."

In the following chapters, the reader will be offered a theoretical and practical model for the enhancement of dentofacial traits through orthodontic treatment. This work should be viewed as a clinical narrative rather than a text or atlas. Its format is intended to first explain the theoretical underpinnings of why patients seek orthodontic treatment and then demonstrate through case analysis practical strategies for achieving successful enhancement of variations in dentofacial traits. When appropriate, I will mention specific technologies and products that I have used in practice. In no way do I have any financial interest in these proprietary goods other than in their ability to aid the practice of enhancement orthodontics. Although all of my patients were treated with fixed labial preadjusted appliances, many of the treatment outcomes could have been achieved by using other appliance types and techniques currently being sold in the orthodontic marketplace.

It is my hope that this book will demystify the nature of orthodontics and enliven the reader's interest in participating in enhancement health care.

Marc Bernard Ackerman
Bryn Mawr, Pennsylvania

Acknowledgments

The enhancement orthodontic concept is based on the contributions of many different individuals in many diverse fields. Progress in any health care specialty is due in large part to the collaborative efforts of clinicians, educators, and researchers. It would be presumptuous for an individual to amalgamate the work of others into a unified model without proper recognition. Grateful acknowledgment is made to the following who have contributed to the development of the enhancement orthodontic model:

Dr. James L. Ackerman, Pittsboro, North Carolina, for his confidence and courage to go against the grain of conventional wisdom in orthodontics for over 45 years. His many publications have laid the groundwork for the enhancement orthodontic concept. On a personal note, he has been a brilliant teacher, partner, editor at large, and father.

Dr. D. Walter Cohen, Philadelphia, Pennsylvania, for his myriad contributions to the profession of dentistry and his pioneering work in the field of periodontal medicine. His unwavering support and belief in my abilities has encouraged me to strive for excellence in my profession.

Dr. Orhan Tuncay, Philadelphia, Pennsylvania, who first motivated me to write this book and who has given me the opportunity to teach these concepts to our residents at Temple University.

Dr. David Sarver, Birmingham, Alabama, who has been a great mentor and writing partner. He is the true "orthodontic missionary," steadfast in advancing new ideas and techniques to a very critical audience.

Dr. Bjorn Zachrisson, Oslo, Norway, whose lectures have elegantly defined and simplified many key appearance concepts in orthodontics.

Dr. Harvey Rosen, Philadelphia, Pennsylvania, for his exceptional skill in performing orthognathic surgery. His work in the field of aesthetic jaw surgery has been revolutionary.

Dr. Robin Harshaw, Bryn Mawr, Pennsylvania, for his compassionate pediatric dental care for two generations of Ackerman orthodontic patients.

Dr. Robert Tisot, Moorestown, New Jersey, for his mentorship and preceptorship, a master clinician whose chair side teaching was unsurpassed.

Dr. Morton Amsterdam, Bala Cynwyd, Pennsylvania, for his development of the Periodontal Prosthesis concept. His tireless efforts enhancing mutilated dentitions that were considered "hopeless" laid the foundation for contemporary advanced restorative dentistry. The idea that variation in occlusal traits can be physiologic was learned by the author in Dr. Amsterdam's seminars.

Thanks are due also to the following for loan of original illustrations:

Dr. D. Walter Cohen
Dr. Harvey Rosen
Imaging Sciences International
Gregory FCA Communications
3dMD (Kelly Duncan)
Interactive Communication and Training (Tom Griffin)

Elsevier Publishing, for permission to reprint material that was recently accepted for publication in the *American Journal of Orthodontics and Dentofacial Orthopedics*.

The entire production staff at Blackwell Publishing deserves recognition, specifically my commissioning editor, Sophia Joyce, and my editor, Erica Judisch, who had confidence in this book from its inception. I would also like to thank all of my patients and my staff at Main Line Orthodontics, without whom this book would not be possible.

Finally, I would like to recognize my entire family for their enduring love and support.

Introduction

I want you to realize that in adopting this specialty you must be something more than a mere mechanic ... You not only make your patient physically better, but you contribute to his self-respect and to his beauty. With limits, you can transform a face from inharmony of feature to symmetry, from ugliness to comeliness, and from a repulsive expression to a winning one. (Norman W. Kingsley, December 3, 1908, in a letter to the Alumni Society of the Angle School of Orthodontia)

Enhancement Orthodontics: Theory and Practice is a radical departure from the conventional approach to orthodontics. In practice, most of our patients are simply seeking improvement of a recognizable variation in a dentofacial trait or mixture of traits and are not necessarily seeking a complete remake of their entire occlusion. A *dentofacial trait* is herein defined as a hard- or soft-tissue characteristic or combination of characteristics, which distinguish an individual's facial appearance and determines their level of oral and social function. Many patients who would have been heretofore classified as within the range of "normal" variation are now asking to go beyond normal. Consequently, present-day orthodontic diagnosis and treatment planning is being driven by the patient and society's *perceptual* and

morphologic ideal rather than a comparative assessment of a patient's anatomy/morphology relative to outdated normative standards. Orthodontic treatment need is best defined by a patient's level of disability arising from variation in dentofacial traits. In order to understand the genesis of this novel orthodontic model, we must first appreciate the conceptual evolution that occurred in the last century of modern orthodontic practice.

Historically, the modern specialty of orthodontics was nurtured in the womb of prosthetic dentistry. In that bygone era, occlusion was the glue that bound the fabric of dentistry together. The intact dentition was the exception rather than the rule and the aspiration of the late nineteenth-century dentist was to create an occlusal scheme for the prosthetic rehabilitation of the mutilated dentition. Perhaps the defining moment in Victorian dentistry was the introduction of Edward Angle's concept of normal occlusion and its application to the natural dentition (Angle 1899). It would largely determine the trajectory of orthodontic theory, research, and practice for the next hundred years.

While Angle's formula was brilliant in its simplicity, it was at the same time severely limited in its one-dimensional classification of the human dentition. More important, Angle and his peers suffered from a type of nineteenth-century fundamentalism, believing that the goal of orthodontic treatment was the attainment of nature's *intended* ideal form. The Achilles heel of Angle's orthodontic model was its total disregard for the ubiquity and normality of human variation. When viewed in light of current knowledge and a century of experience, we recognize that nature in no way intends for the orthodontist to achieve perfection, but rather it often grapples with the orthodontist trying to achieve perfection. Nature imposes a series of limitations on the orthodontist's ability to modify any given dentofacial trait. Norman W. Kingsley, the predecessor of Angle and the "father of orthodontia," concluded, "The perversity and contrariness of inanimate things is proverbial and nowhere more strikingly exhibited than in the effort of Nature, when forcibly diverted, to return to its former condition" (Kingsley 1908).

The vast majority of orthodontic research efforts through the latter part of the twentieth century focused primarily on understanding "normal" growth of the craniofacial skeleton and the skeletal hard-tissue limitations affecting orthodontic treatment. It was postulated that if orthodontists could understand the sequence and timing of craniofacial growth and development, then they could appropriately time the application of mechanical devices to alter, augment, and even reverse any hard-tissue deviation from "normal." Recent randomized clinical trials in orthodontics have demonstrated that although growth modification therapy can elicit clinically detectable change in the short term, there is no evidence that it is maintained in the long term (Wheeler et al. 2002, Tulloch et al. 2004).

In essence, orthodontists have learned that it is really the soft tissues that regulate therapeutic modifiability in orthodontic treatment (Ackerman et al. 1999). Several aspects related to soft-tissue form and function largely determine the boundaries of dental compensation for an underlying skeletal problem, that is, the pressures exerted by the lips, cheeks, and tongue on the teeth, the periodontal attachment apparatus, the muscles and connective tissue components of the temporomandibular joint, and the contours of the integument of the face. Thus, the clinician's goal in orthodontic diagnosis and treatment planning has been to discern the patient's limits of soft-tissue adaptation, relative to the dental and skeletal changes needed to satisfy their desired dentofacial outcome. The extent to which the patient's morphology varies from their perceived ideal will determine whether or not orthodontics alone or orthodontics in combination with other modalities will be needed to fulfill their expectations of treatment.

Today, the role of the clinician engaged in the practice of orthodontics is to act as the change agent for enhancement of dentofacial traits. When viewed in this context, any treatment rendered will be based on patient-directed objectives. Orthodontists are neither occlusionists nor estheticians; they are merely health professionals with the ability to enhance a recognizable variation in a dentofacial trait or mixture of traits, improving the health and wellness of their patients.

REFERENCES

Ackerman, J.L., Proffit, W.R., Sarver, D.M. 1999. The emerging soft tissue paradigm in orthodontic diagnosis and treatment planning. *Clin Orth Res* 2:49–52.

Angle, E.H. 1899. Classification of malocclusion. *Dental Cosmos* 41:248–264, 350–357.

Kingsley, N.W. 1908. A letter to the Alumni Society of the Angle School of Orthodontia. *American Orthodontist*, p. 125.

Tulloch, J.F.C., Proffit, W.R., Phillips, C. 2004. Outcomes in a 2-phase randomized clinical trial of early Class II treatment. *Am J Orthod Dentofac Orthop* 125:657–667.

Wheeler, T.T., McGorray, S.P., Dolce, C., Taylor, M.G., King, G.J. 2002. Effectiveness of early treatment of Class II malocclusion. *Am J Orthod Dentofac Orthop* 121:9–17.

Theory

Orthodontics Defined

1

The primary goal for most patients seeking orthodontic treatment is a discernible improvement in some aspect of his or her dentofacial appearance. Orthodontic therapy, to their way of thinking, is something that makes you look better and feel better about yourself and perhaps enhances your ability to socially interact with others (e.g., to find a mate or make an impression with a potential employer). The dental profession has fostered the notion that enhanced occlusion improves the health and longevity of the dentition, so in effect many patients seeking orthodontic care state that their secondary goal of treatment is an oral health benefit. Thus, there is a significant disparity between the end-user and the health provider's perception of what drives orthodontic need. The goal of this chapter is to define orthodontics relative to health and to describe the needs of our specialty's intended end-user, the patient.

The Medicalization of Orthodontics

There has been an increasing trend in our society to view naturally occurring biological processes, such as menopause, as ailments or illnesses. As such, these phenomena are incorporated into medical practice with various treatments, such as hormone replacement therapy prescribed for a vast number of healthy women. In some instances, such as alcoholism ("drunkards" are now considered to have an illness), this trend is undoubtedly enlightened, yet in other cases, such as treating skin wrinkling during aging as an ailment, this trend is highly suspect, particularly because the "problem" affects every man and woman in the world. This trend has been called *medicalization,* and there is a concern that the sphere of medical practice is enlarging to include entities that do not legitimately deserve to be part of medical practice. In some ways the notion that any deviation in occlusion from the theoretical ideal is abnormal represents medicalization of naturally occurring morphologic variation. *Medicalization* is "the tendency to conceive an activity, phenomenon, behavior, condition, etc., as a disease or disorder or as an affliction that should be regarded as a disease or disorder: 1) people suffer it (patienthood); 2) the causes are physical and somatic not psychic; 3) it requires and demands treatment aimed at cure or relief of symptoms; 4) at the hands of persons licensed in the healing arts; and

5) this conception of the condition will be supported by society out of interest in the health of its people" (The President's Council on Bioethics 2003). The traditional approach of classifying malocclusion is a type of medicalization. The medicalized model of orthodontics is based on the theory that normal occlusion is *the* essential requirement for orthodontic health.

The assumption is that there is a universal standard of *dentofacial normality* and, in particular, one ideal occlusal scheme (constellation of dental traits) naturally occurring in the species, which is correlated with superior oral health, function, and appearance. Orthodontic health has been measured relative to the amount of divergence from a Class I molar relationship with the mesiobuccal cusp of the maxillary first molar in the buccal groove of the mandibular first molar, the teeth within the arches aligned on a line of occlusion, and very little overbite and overjet (Angle 1899). *Malocclusion*, in the orthodontic disease construct, refers to *any* deviation of the teeth from ideal occlusion. Unfortunately, *ideal occlusion* has been used synonymously with the term *normal occlusion*.

It has been postulated that deviations from ideal occlusion have a causal relationship with both dental decay and periodontal disease. Many clinicians argue that it is easier to clean straight teeth (or those with ideal occlusion) than to clean "crooked" teeth. However, recent data suggest that an individual's willingness and motivation for maintaining oral hygiene have a greater impact on dental disease than does how well teeth are aligned. That is, the effect of variation in tooth alignment on dental disease is less important than the patient's oral hygiene status (Helm and Peterson 1989).

Several studies in the late 1970s that examined a large number of orthodontically treated patients 10 to 20 years post treatment provide some data on long-term relationships between deviations from ideal occlusion and oral health (Sadowsky and BeGole 1981, Polson et al. 1988). In both studies, a comparison of patients who underwent orthodontic treatment with untreated individuals in the same age group demonstrated a similar periodontal status, despite the ideal type occlusions of the orthodontically treated group. There was no evidence of a beneficial effect of orthodontic treatment on future periodontal health. In addition, routine orthodontic treatment does not appear to have an iatrogenic effect on the periodontium. Long-term studies demonstrate that physiologically sound orthodontic treatment does not increase the likelihood of later periodontal manifestations. Although case reports illustrating the effects of nonphysiologic orthodontic treatment exist in the literature, there are no well-controlled prospective studies regarding the predictability of the periodontal tissue response to any given orthodontic treatment.

It has also been suggested by some dentists that even minor deviations from ideal occlusion will trigger parafunctional habits such as bruxism and clenching. If this indeed were the case, most individuals' occlusions would need treatment to prevent the development of pain in the masticatory muscles. Data suggest that because a large portion of the population has moderate deviation from ideal occlusion (roughly 50–75%) and this number far exceeds the amount of the population with temporomandibular joint dysfunction (TMD) (5–30%, depending on the symptoms examined), it seems unlikely that variation in occlusion alone is the cause of hyperactivity of the masticatory muscles associated with the temporomandibular joint (Greene 1995). In summary, occlusion (Huang 2004), condyle position, and orthodontic treatment (Gianelly 1989) have not been demonstrated to cause TMD.

The last warmly held notion regarding ideal occlusion concerns facial appearance. It has been thought that the most functional arrangement of the teeth along their lines of occlusion produces the most attractive faces. In the absence of an underlying skeletal disproportion or tooth size/arch size

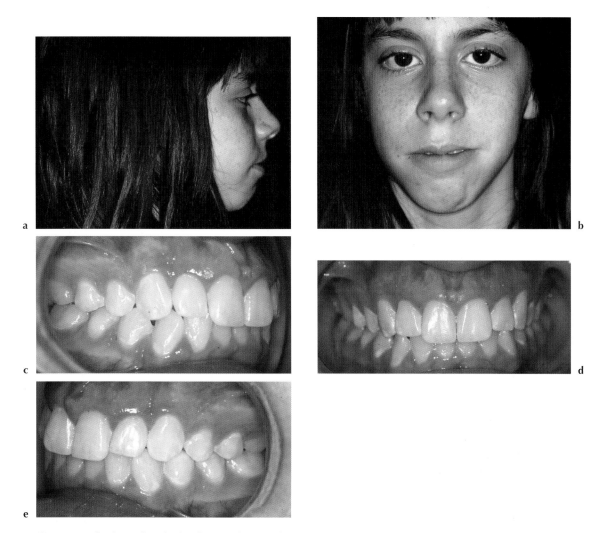

Figure 1.1 It has been thought that the most functional arrangement of the teeth along their lines of occlusion produces the most attractive faces. In the absence of an underlying skeletal disproportion or tooth size–arch size discrepancy, this hypothesis usually holds true. However, when there is an anteroposterior or vertical skeletal discrepancy or excessive tooth mass relative to arch perimeter, the orthodontic tooth movement needed to achieve ideal occlusion has to compensate for that disproportion, which results in dental expansion beyond the limits of the soft-tissue envelope and, consequently, compromised facial appearance. Although this patient has a near-ideal type occlusion, her facial appearance is negatively affected by lip incompetence, a long lower facial height, and a convex/posteriorly divergent profile (**A–E**).

discrepancy, this hypothesis usually holds true. However, when there is an anteroposterior or a vertical skeletal discrepancy or excessive tooth mass relative to arch perimeter, the orthodontic tooth movement needed to achieve ideal occlusion has to compensate for that disproportion, which results in dental expansion beyond the limits of the soft-tissue envelope and, consequently, compromised facial appearance (Fig. 1.1).

A more biologically valid concept of normal (ideal) occlusion would include a range of variation in the relevant dental traits that are compatible with facial appearance and unimpaired oral function. It is currently impossible to determine the point at which normal variation in many dentofacial traits becomes abnormal or induces pathologic function. The clinician must consider a patient's occlusion as one ingredient in the recipe for orthodontic health. Ideal occlusion is a good starting point for assessment of a patient's occlusion but not a practical end point for *all* patients. Unless variation in a patient's occlusion has a direct effect on the patient, dentists should no longer use it as the "medical" reason for orthodontic treatment.

Psychosocial Considerations

Well-aligned teeth and a pleasing smile afford positive social status, whereas irregular or protruding teeth are attached to negative status (Shaw 1981, Shaw et al. 1985). As well, there is a linear relationship between straight teeth and judgments about intelligence, sincerity, and conscientiousness (Linn 1966). Children with severe variation in dental traits have the greatest desire for orthodontic treatment, although there is no difference in motivation for treatment between children with moderate variation in dental traits and those with "normal" dental traits (Lewit and Virolainen 1968). In a clinic population, it is the mother who often is the deciding and motivating factor for seeking orthodontic treatment for her children. Parental assessment of orthodontic treatment need is related more to social factors (improvement in status) than to objective evidence of the severity of the problem (Baldwin and Barnes 1965).

Orthodontic Handicap Defined

In the early 1970s, the Office of the Surgeon General, United States Army, asked the National Academy of Sciences–National Research Council to recommend for use in military health care programs a definition of orthodontic conditions that are seriously handicapping and to recommend objective clinical criteria for describing those conditions. The Army's desire for such advice came from the directives that regulated orthodontic care for eligible military dependents *only* if the condition being treated was seriously physically handicapping. The Committee on Handicapping Orthodontic Conditions (CHOC) was formed to address the questions of what constitutes an orthodontic handicap and who should qualify for orthodontic treatment. In their final report (The National Research Council 1976), the CHOC defined a "handicapping orthodontic condition" as:

A clinically obvious physical abnormality of tooth and/or jaw relationships. It results in disability characterized by physical, emotional, and social dysfunction. The measure of a person's degree of handicap is the extent to which his disability affects him. Thus, a seriously handicapping orthodontic condition is a dentofacial abnormality that severely compromises a person's physical or emotional health. Physical health is severely compromised if disability of the oral function of breathing, speaking, or eating accompanies the abnormality, especially if tissue destruction is occurring. Emotional health is severely compromised if the abnormality causes others to react negatively, so that the person is treated differently by his peers because of the abnormality, or if the abnormality causes his self-image and self-esteem to be affected to such an extent that his life adjustment is altered.

The CHOC concluded that a relatively small percentage (14%) of the pediatric population had *seriously* handicapping orthodontic conditions (The National Research Council 1976). However, the CHOC recommended that a range of handicapping orthodontic conditions should qualify for either partial or full coverage under the military and civilian health benefit.

By incorporating elements of physical, mental, and social well-being into the definition of orthodontic need, the handicapping condition approach broadened the scope of orthodontics to include psychosocial factors that had been previously excluded from clinical assessment. The demand for orthodontic intervention hinges on an individual's level of physical and emotional disability. Unfortunately, this view of orthodontic need was never adopted into general clinical practice or health care policy. However, it introduced the concept of treatment need being a function of individual handicap in the social context.

Bioethical Perspective: Enhancement Versus Therapy

As more and more patients are seeking elective medical and dental treatments largely aimed at improvement of their appearance and physical fitness, bioethicists have raised questions related to the morality of providing this type of health care (The President's Council on Bioethics 2003). Historically, the primary role of the physician or dentist was to act as a "healer" of the sick. The goal of *therapy* in medicine and dentistry has traditionally been to treat individuals with known diseases, disabilities, or impairments, in order to restore them to a normal state of health and fitness. The goal of *enhancement* in contemporary medicine and dentistry has been to alter the "normal" state of the individual's body or mind in order to augment or improve his or her inherent capacities and physical/social functioning. Bioethicists, to distinguish between morally acceptable and unacceptable clinical interventions, introduced this contradistinction between therapy and enhancement. Essentially, it was initially thought that those interventions characterized as "therapy" are ethically agreeable and those interventions characterized as "enhancement" are ethically suspect. For example, gene therapy to cure multiple sclerosis is acceptable. However, gene therapy to increase height in a person who is unhappy with their short stature is suspect.

Although the distinction between therapy and enhancement calls attention to this moral problem facing practitioners of orthodontics, it is still ambiguous and not entirely practical for clinical application. Enhancement by definition generally signifies a quantitative change, an increase in magnitude or degree. It is quite subjective and abstract relative to moral judgments. More important, therapy and enhancement are overlapping categorizations. *All* therapies with successful outcomes are enhancing, even though not all enhancements with successful outcomes are therapeutic. The central problem in separating enhancement from therapy is that they are both inextricably linked to the intrinsic difficulty in defining health and the concept of normality.

Defining Health

The World Health Organization (WHO) defines *health* as "a state of complete physical, mental, and social well being and not merely the absence of disease or infirmity" (WHO 1946). When viewed in the context of this definition of health, any medical or dental intervention directed at the enhancement of an individual's physical, mental, or social well-being may be considered part of health promotion and therapeutic in nature. In the hope of clinicians using a standard language and conceptual framework for the description of health, the WHO created the *International Classification of Functioning, Disability and Health (ICF)* (WHO 2001). The ICF provides a basis for definition, measurement, and public policy decisions related to health and disability. In the past, disability began where health ended, and consequently once one was labeled as disabled, the focus became one's level of dysfunction rather than one's level of health. The ICF recognizes that every human being can and will experience a decrement in health and, as a result, will experience some disability. By shifting the focus from the etiology of disability to the impact disability has on the individual, the ICF places *all* health conditions on an equal plane, allowing them to be compared along the lines of health and disability (WHO 2002).

Defining Disability

Historically, there have been two conceptual models of disability. The *medical model* regards disability as an inherent aspect of the individual, directly caused by disease or other health condition, which demands medical intervention in the form of treatment by professionals. Disability in this model requires medical treatment to "correct" the problem with the individual. The *social model* regards disability as a socially created problem and not an inherent aspect of the individual. In this model, disability requires a societal response because an adverse physical environment stemming from attitudes of the society has created the problem. Each model partially describes the complex nature of disability. In all cases, disability describes the interaction between attributes of a person and attributes of the overall context in which the person lives. To wit, there are internal components (medical) and external components (social) of disability. Synthesizing the core features of these two models, the ICF offers a more useful model of disability termed the *biopsychosocial model*.

The biopsychosocial model of health and disability (WHO 2002) incorporates the three different perspectives of health: biological, individual, and social (Fig. 1.2).

Disability and functioning are predicated on the interactions between an individual's health condition(s) and contextual factors. The contextual factors include both external environmental elements (e.g., social attitudes) and internal personal elements (e.g., gender, age, social background, past and present experience, etc.), which can influence how the individual experiences disability. Essentially, there are three levels of function-

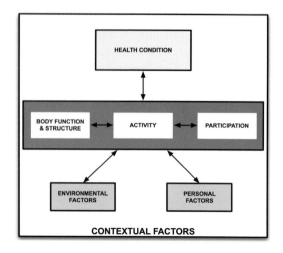

Figure 1.2 The biopsychosocial model of health and disability. (Adapted from The World Health Organization. 2002. *Towards a common language for functioning, disability, and health: ICF.* Geneva, Switzerland: World Health Organization.)

ing classified by the ICF. First, there is functioning at the level of the body part or parts. Second, there is functioning of the whole person. Third, there is functioning of the whole person in a social context. Disability involves dysfunction at one or more of these levels causing impairments, activity limitations, and participation restrictions. The formal definitions of key terminology in the ICF are listed below (WHO 2002):

- *Body functions* are physiologic functions of body systems (including psychological functions).
- *Body structures* are anatomical parts of the body such as organs, limbs, and their components.
- *Impairments* are problems in body function or structure such as a significant deviation or loss.
- *Activity* is the execution of a task or an action by an individual.
- *Activity limitations* are difficulties an individual may have in executing activities.
- *Participation restrictions* are problems an individual may experience in involvement in life situations.

Table 1.1 Orthodontic conditions and their effect on health and disability.

Orthodontic Condition	Impairment	Activity Limitation	Participation Restriction
Cleft lip and palate	Mastication, Speech	Difficulty in eating and communication	Poor speech can lead to teasing and negative performance in school
Severe anterior open bite	Difficulty incising	Avoidance of certain foods	Social stigma associated with altered chewing
Missing anterior tooth	Appearance disfigurement	None	Avoidance of smiling due to negative reaction of others
Mottled enamel	None	Reluctance to smile	Can seem unfriendly making it more difficult to establish friendships
Protruding incisors	None	None	Teased by peers
Posterior crossbite with no mandibular deflection	None	None	None

- *Environmental factors* make up the physical, social, and attitudinal environment in which people live and conduct their lives.

Orthodontics Defined

Orthodontics is the specialized branch of dentistry concerned with variations in dentofacial traits that may affect an individual's overall well-being. A *dentofacial trait* is defined as a hard or soft tissue characteristic or combination of characteristics that distinguish an individual's facial appearance and determines his or her level of oral and social function. *Orthodontic health* is defined as a constellation of dentofacial traits consistent with a state of complete physical, mental, and social well-being; that is, the absence of impairment, activity limitation, and participation restriction. Orthodontic intervention includes therapies that enhance a dentofacial trait or traits, thus improving a person's level of health (wellness). An orthodontist must recognize hard and soft tissue limitations imposed by human variation and communicate to the patient the extent to which orthodontics alone or in combination with other modalities of treatment may modify a dentofacial trait or traits.

Practical Application

If an orthodontic condition is clinically detected by the doctor or perceived by the patient, it must be assessed relative to the patient's three levels of functioning: body part(s), whole person, and the individual in the context of societal values. A diagnosis of a reduction in the individual's state of orthodontic health is determined by the extent of impairment, activity limitation, or participation restriction linked to the specific variation in their dentofacial trait(s) (Table 1.1).

The clinical examples in Table 1.1 illustrate that different potential orthodontic conditions have specific effects stretching across one, two, or three levels of disability. As a result, there are different levels of intervention linked to the three different levels of orthodontic disability (Table 1.2).

All orthodontic interventions should improve a patient's state of health while at the same time diminishing the extent of their disability.

The Future of Orthodontics

Peer-reviewed journals have recently initiated a call for evidence-based systematic reviews in order to summarize the large

Table 1.2 The levels of orthodontic disability and the potential levels of intervention.

Level of Orthodontic Disability	Level of Intervention
Impairment (*body part*)	Evaluation Orthodontic treatment Potential referral to other specialties if appropriate
Activity limitation (*whole person*)	Evaluation Orthodontic treatment Potential referral to other specialties if appropriate Counseling
Participation restriction (*individual-societal context*)	Evaluation Orthodontic treatment Potential referral to other specialties if appropriate Counseling Improved access to orthodontic treatment (societal level) Public education about variation in dentofacial traits (societal level) Public education about orthodontic treatment (societal level)

Participation restriction is usually a result of societal attitudes, and intervention is directed at both the general public and the individual.

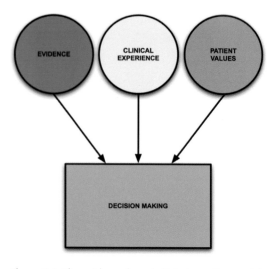

Figure 1.3 The evidence-based clinical practice model.

amount of literature that clinicians need to assimilate into practice. Scientific studies are weighted based on their vulnerability to bias. The hierarchy of evidence for therapeutic interventions listed in ascending order of bias are randomized controlled clinical trials, nonrandomized controlled clinical trials, cohort studies, case-control studies, crossover studies, cross-sectional studies, case studies, and consensus reports reflecting the opinions of experts in a given field. For the most part, medicine and dentistry as a whole have embraced the systematic review of the literature and have begun to utilize evidence-based strategies to educate current and future clinicians.

In the evidence-based clinical practice (EBCP) model, there are three elements required for the provision of evidence-based care. First, the clinician must integrate the best scientific evidence available into the decision-making process. Second, the clinician must apply his or her accrued clinical experience to the decision-making process. Third, the clinician must appreciate the *patient's preferences* as they relate to their treatment need(s) and assimilate this into the decision-making process (Ismail and Bader 2004) (Fig. 1.3).

The EBCP model indicates whether to apply interventions and which specific interventions to apply based on weighing benefits and risks, inconvenience, and costs within the context of patient values.

The difficulties in applying EBCP to orthodontics have been threefold. First, the vast majority of literature in the specialty contains a great deal of bias (poor study design) and is focused on the "how-to perform" orthodontic treatment rather than the "why to perform" orthodontic treatment. Second, the amount of literature in the specialty regarding patient preferences is small. Third, there is currently no consensus in the specialty as to the definition of *orthodontic health* and consequently the definition of *orthodontic need*. The net effect of these problems has been limited use and great skepticism of EBCP.

Decision-making in clinical practice is not based wholly on evidence or experience. It is based on practical reasoning called *clinical judgment*. Opponents in the current debate would agree that the hallmark of a good orthodontist is the capacity to exercise sound clinical judgment. This essential skill incorporates application of experience and scrutiny of evidence, complementary properties compatible in, and necessary for, interpretative reasoning. Clinical judgment determines what is optimal for that individual at the time when the only available evidence is extracted from averages. It is perception based on experience with sometimes-scant scientific evidence to support it. Scientific evidence alone may reduce, but not eliminate, uncertainty when making clinical decisions or predicting outcomes, but clinical judgment refined by experience is essential for sound clinical decision-making.

In orthodontic practice, clinical judgment involves an integration of clinical experience and a systematic assessment of relevant scientific evidence in the context of the patient's orthodontic condition, treatment needs, and preferences. Clinical judgment is a skill (*art*), using the best available evidence (*science*) with societal and patient values (*trans-science*) (Ackerman 1974). Overall, the proper method of clinical practice is reflective, experienced evidence-bolstered orthodontics (Ackerman et al. 2006).

The future of orthodontics will require new and innovative research to develop a clinical database elucidating the factors governing orthodontic health and disability. Orthodontists have plenty of mechanical experience; we merely need to focus more on our patients' preferences and how society views our profession. In the interim, the focus should be on improved communication with our patients in order to provide the enhancements they are seeking.

REFERENCES

Ackerman, J.L. 1974. Orthodontics: Art, science, or trans-science? *Angle Orthod* 44:243–250.

Ackerman, J.L., Kean, M.R., Ackerman, M.B. 2006. Evidence-bolstered orthodontics. *Austral Orthod J* 22:69–70.

Ackerman, M. 2004. Evidence-based orthodontics for the 21st century. *J Am Dent Assoc* 135:162–167.

Angle, E.H. 1899. Classification of malocclusion. *Dental Cosmos* 41:248–264, 350–357.

Baldwin, D.C., Jr., Barnes, M.L. 1965. Psychosocial factors motivating orthodontic treatment. *Int Assoc Dental Res Meeting* 43:153 (abstract).

Gianelly, A.A. 1989. Orthodontics, condylar position and TMJ status. *Am J Orthod Dentofac Orthop* 75:521–523.

Greene, C.S. 1995. Etiology of temporomandibular disorders. *Semin Orthod* 1:222–228.

Helm, S., Peterson, P.E. 1989. Causal relation between malocclusion and caries. *Acta Odontol Scand* 47:217–221.

Huang, G. 2004. Occlusal adjustment for treating and preventing temporomandibular disorders. *Am J Orthod Dentofac Orthod* 126:138–139.

Ismail, A., Bader, J.D. 2004. Evidence-based dentistry in clinical practice. *J Am Dent Assoc* 135:78–83.

Lewit, D.W., Virolainen, K. 1968. Conformity and independence in adolescents' motivation for orthodontic treatment. *Child Develop* 39:1189–1200.

Linn, E.L. 1966. Social meanings of dental appearance. *J Health Human Behav* 7:289–295.

Polson, A.M., Subtelny, J.D., Meitner, S.W., Polson, A.P., Sommers, E.W., Iker, H.P., Reed, B.E. 1988. Long-term periodontal status after orthodontic treatment. *Am J Orthod Dentofac Orthop* 93:51–58.

Sadowsky, C., BeGole, E.A. 1981. Long-term effects of orthodontic treatment on periodontal health. *Am J Orthod* 80:156–172.

Shaw, W.C. 1981. The influence of children's dentofacial appearance on their social attractiveness as judged by peers and lay adults. *Am J Orthod* 79:399–415.

Shaw, W.C., Rees, G., Dawe, M., Charles, C.R. 1985. The influence of dentofacial appearance on the social attractiveness of young adults. *Am J Orthod* 87:21–26.

The National Research Council. 1976. *Seriously handicapping orthodontic conditions.* Washington, D.C.: National Academy of Sciences.

The President's Council on Bioethics. 2003. *Beyond therapy: Biotechnology and the pursuit of happiness.* Washington, D.C.: President's Council on Bioethics.

The World Health Organization. 1946. *Preamble to the Constitution of the World Health Organization as adopted by the International Health Conference,* New York, 19–22 June, 1946; signed on 22 July 1946 by the representatives of 61 states (official records of the World Health Organization, No. 2, p. 100) and entered into force on 7 April 1948.

The World Health Organization. 2001. *International classification of functioning, disability, and health.* Geneva, Switzerland: World Health Organization.

The World Health Organization. 2002. *Towards a common language for functioning, disability, and health: ICF.* Geneva, Switzerland: World Health Organization.

Communication in Orthodontics

2

One of today's greatest challenges in orthodontics is the acceptance of the ethical imperative that empowers the patient or patient's parents to serve as full partners in the decision-making process. Long gone are the paternalistic days of "the doctor knows best." The resultant dilemma for dentists is to balance advocacy for a patient's potentially ideal orthodontic outcome while respecting the patient's right to self-determination, which might entail a lower expectation of orthodontic intervention. Self-determination in this context is an individual's right to control what happens to his or her body. Thus, the conflict for the orthodontist comes from wanting to perform the highest level of orthodontics possible while at the same time complying with the patient's right to decide on what treatment alternative is best suited to his or her needs. From a medicolegal standpoint as well as a treatment outcome point of view, the doctor must initiate a dialogue with the patient or parent of the patient in order to jointly construct a treatment plan that satisfies all parties involved. The goal of this chapter is to offer a strategy for successful communication with patients (and/or their parents) seeking orthodontic treatment.

Strategy for Successful Communication in Orthodontics

Initial Patient Contact

Communication with the orthodontic patient often begins with the call to the office to schedule an initial examination appointment. The receptionist or treatment coordinator should record important demographic information about the patient during this telephone conversation. They should ask for the patient's age, address, dentist, source of referral, and, if known, reason for referral (Fig. 2.1).

The responses will help the orthodontist prepare the appropriate line of questioning at the time of the initial examination. For example, an orthodontist can often gauge the patient's level of orthodontic awareness based on how many other patients they treat in that patient's neighborhood. They may also get a sense for the patient's orthodontic awareness by knowing who referred the patient to the office. Referring dentists in the area may have a specific referral pattern based on their own orthodontic knowledge base and level of clinical experience. The ease or difficulty

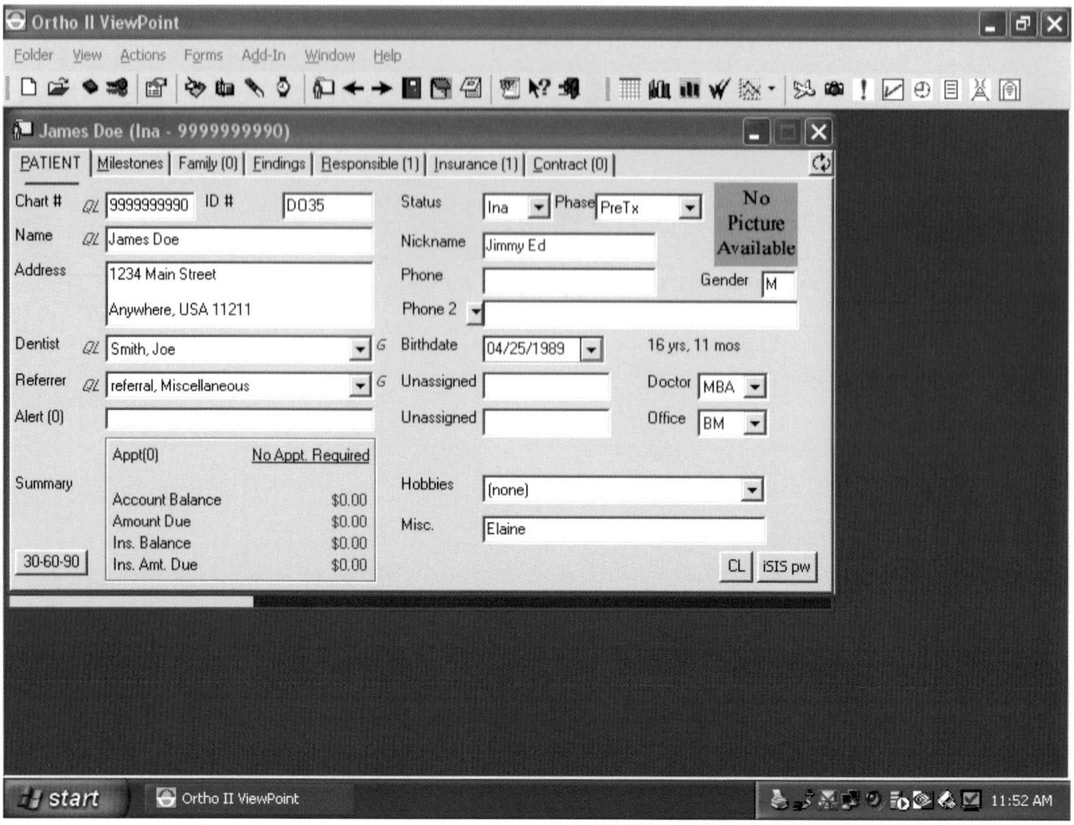

a

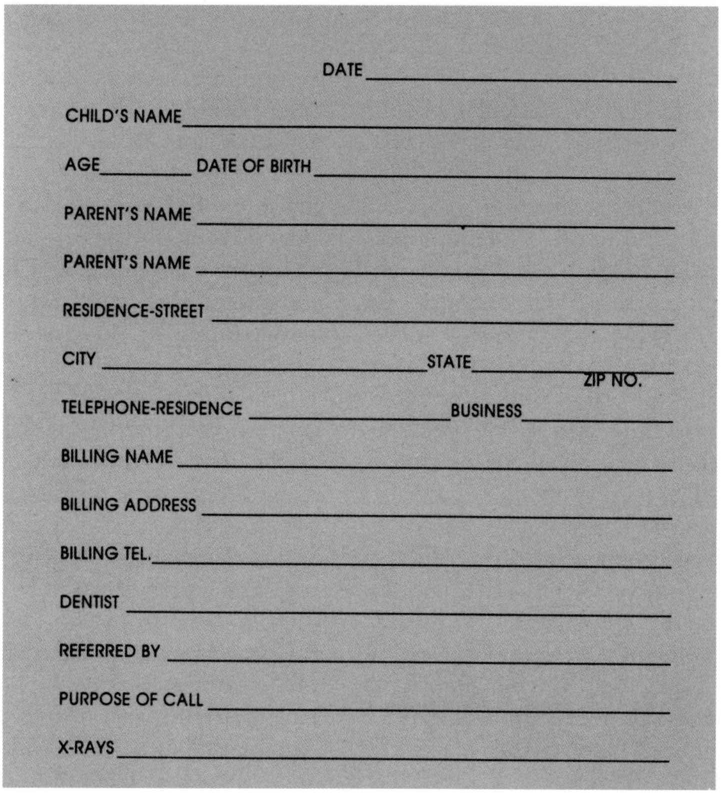

DATE _____

CHILD'S NAME _____

AGE _____ DATE OF BIRTH _____

PARENT'S NAME _____

PARENT'S NAME _____

RESIDENCE-STREET _____

CITY _____ STATE _____
ZIP NO. _____

TELEPHONE-RESIDENCE _____ BUSINESS _____

BILLING NAME _____

BILLING ADDRESS _____

BILLING TEL. _____

DENTIST _____

REFERRED BY _____

PURPOSE OF CALL _____

X-RAYS _____

b

Figure 2.1 (**A**) Orthodontic practice management software allows the clinician to create electronic patient records and establish a database of demographic information. (Screen image from Ortho II Viewpoint Software, Ames, Iowa.) (**B**) New patient telephone calls can also be recorded on a paper form and then transferred to the computer at the time of the initial examination appointment.

with which the staff can schedule the initial examination will indicate how demanding this patient or parent may be in the future and perhaps how much cooperation can be expected during active treatment. In the author's practice, the staff member concludes the telephone conversation by explaining to the patient or parent what occurs during the initial examination. They are told that they will receive, via mail, a personalized health questionnaire with a preaddressed, stamped envelope that they should return prior to the visit (Fig. 2.2).

The Health Questionnaire

The primary purpose of the health questionnaire in orthodontics is to help determine a patient's level of well-being. In keeping with the World Health Organization's definition of *health* (see Chapter 1), this instrument should attempt to elicit the status of the patient's physical, mental, and social well-being. The component parts of the health questionnaire are the patient's chief concern, psychosocial status, growth status (if a child or an adolescent), dental history, and medical history. A thorough review of the health questionnaire should be undertaken before meeting with the patient and/or parent.

Chief Concern

There are several reasons why patients seek an orthodontic evaluation. As discussed earlier, the patient may have a negative awareness of a recognizable variation in a dentofacial trait or traits. Less frequently, the patient may have a detectable impairment in oral function. However, one of the more common reasons for patient referral is "my dentist said that I need braces." It is helpful to ascertain whether the patient is seeking information, immediate treatment, clarification of previously received information, or conflicting information. In any of these cases, the orthodontist should be prepared to further discuss the nature of the

chief concern with the patient at the initial examination.

Psychosocial Status

The patient's social and behavioral history is exceedingly important as it relates to his or her motivation for seeking orthodontic treatment and his or her expectation of orthodontic treatment. As well, the patient's behavioral history is a good predictor of the patient's ability to cooperate. The approach to discerning a patient's psychosocial status depends on whether the patient is a child, an adolescent, or an adult.

The child or adolescent orthodontic patient's motivation for treatment is either external or internal. External motivation is usually determined by pressure from another individual. An example of an external motivator is a mother who brings her child for an orthodontic evaluation because she is unhappy with the child's dentofacial appearance. Internal motivation is derived from within the individual and is based on the individual's self-concept and perceived need for treatment. It is rare to find a child or adolescent patient with purely internal motivation. However, it is important that at some level they place importance on the treatment being performed. Perhaps the most important question for the parent on the health history is, "Does the child or adolescent recognize a need for treatment?" In terms of cooperation, the child or adolescent who feels that treatment is being done *for* them rather than *to* them will be much more receptive to the orthodontist's demands. The health questionnaire should ask open-ended questions about any disability related to emotional or learning problems. Parents will usually be quite open about a child or an adolescent's school performance at both the academic and social levels.

As far as adult patients, the social history should ascertain information about their emotional wellness and their expectations of treatment. If the patient indicates that he or she is under the care of a psychologist or

PATIENT and PARENT INFORMATION
Please verify and complete information

April 9, 2006
ID# 9999999990
Name/Sex: James Edward Doe, Jr.   Nickname: Jimmy Ed   M
School: _____ Grade: _____
Birth Date/Age: April 25, 1989 16 yrs. 11 mos.
Patient Address: 1234 Main Street
City, State, Zip: Anywhere, USA 11211
Patient Home Phone: email:
Billing Name: Mr. & Mrs. James Edward Doe, Sr.
Spouse Name: Mary   Marital Status: Married
Billing Address: 1234 Main Street
Billing City, State, Zip: Anywhere, USA 11211
Billing Phone:
General Dentist or Pedodontist: Dr. Joe Smith
Address: 1 Elm Street , Bryn Mawr, PA 19010
Date of last dental exam:_____ Results:_____
Referred by: Dr. Joe Smith
Mother's Employer:_____ Business Phone_____
Occupation:_____ No. of years employed:_____
Father's Employer:_____ Business Phone_____
Occupation:_____ No. of years employed:_____
Has any other family member been seen by Dr. Ackerman? _____
Names and ages of other children in family: _____

PSYCHOSOCIAL AND PHYSICAL GROWTH STATUS

Jimmy Ed's Chief Concern: _____

Reason for seeking orthodontic advice:

[ ] Information
[ ] Treatment at this time
[ ] Clarification of previously received information or conflicting information
[ ] Continuation of treatment

Does Jimmy Ed have an emotional or nervous problem? Yes__ No__

Is Jimmy Ed learning or physically challenged? _____

Is it likely that Jimmy Ed will be an early maturer or a later maturer physically?
Average___ Early___ Late___

Has Jimmy Ed reached puberty? Yes__ No__
(Females – started menstruation; Males – voice changed)

Is there any significant family history of jaw or teeth problems? Yes__ No__
If yes, please elaborate:_____

Has either parent had orthodontic treatment? Yes__ No__

Are you interested in improving the appearance of Jimmy Ed's teeth at this time even though additional treatment will be needed later? Yes__ No__

a   Does Jimmy Ed recognize a need for orthodontic treatment? Yes__ No__

Figure 2.2 (**A**, **B**) The Orthodontic Health Questionnaire.

MEDICAL/DENTAL HISTORY

Please fill in Medical History for Jimmy Ed

Does Jimmy Ed have a health problem? Yes___ No___

Does Jimmy Ed have a history of major illness? Yes___ No___

Has Jimmy Ed been under the care of a physician for illness recently? Yes___ No___
Please list:_____

Have tonsils and adenoids been removed? Yes___ No___   What age? ____

List any drugs or medications now being taken and give reasons:
_____

List any allergies or drug sensitivities:_____

Has Jimmy Ed ever had surgery? Yes___ No___
Please list:_____

Does Jimmy Ed bleed excessively when cut? Yes___ No___

Jimmy Ed's physician: _____
Date of last physical exam_____ Results:_____

Has Jimmy Ed had any injuries to the face, mouth, or teeth? Yes___ No___

Has Jimmy Ed ever sucked a thumb or fingers? Yes___ No___   What age?____

Circle any of the following for which Jimmy Ed has been treated:

Pneumonia	Anemia	Prolonged bleeding
Heart trouble	Epilepsy	Nervous disorders
Rheumatic fever	Asthma	Liver involvements
Bone disorders	Kidney involvement	Convulsions
Thyroid problems	Speech problems	Cerebral Palsy
Chronic Sinusitis	Hearing problems	Lunch problems
School problems	Malignancies	Measles
Chicken pox	Mumps	AIDS or HIV infection
Hemophilia	Hepatitis	Fainting or dizziness
Diabetes	Tuberculosis	Endocrine problems
Eating disorder	G.E. Reflux	

b Signature   **Relationship to patient**

Figure 2.2 *Continued*

psychiatrist, the orthodontist should ask permission to speak with the mental health provider. If the adult patient is seeking an elective and purely cosmetic enhancement of a dentofacial trait or traits, it is important that the orthodontist evaluate the motivation for doing so. If the patient seeks treatment to merely look better, he or she has a reasonable expectation of treatment. If, on the other hand, the patient thinks that he or she will automatically land a better job after orthodontic treatment, they have an unreasonable expectation of treatment.

Growth Status

In the growing patient seeking orthodontic treatment, it is important to assess physical growth status. The key question is where the patient stands relative to the onset of the adolescent growth phase. Adolescence is defined as the period of life when children reach sexual maturity. It is a transitional period between childhood and adulthood during which the individual attains secondary sex characteristics, undergoes the puberal growth spurt, and achieves fertility and major physiologic changes take place.

On average, the adolescent growth phase occurs 2 years earlier in girls than in boys (Marshall and Tanner 1986). Although there is a great amount of individual variation, the secondary sex characteristics provide a timeline of adolescence for the individual patient. In girls, there are three stages of adolescence. The first stage, which marks the beginning of the puberal growth spurt, is the emergence of the breast buds. The peak velocity of physical growth occurs about 1 year after the initiation of stage 1 and coincides with stage 2. Stage 2 is characterized by well-defined breast development and the presence of both pubic and underarm hair. The third and last stage is marked by the onset of menarche, which occurs roughly 1 to $1\frac{1}{2}$ years after stage 2. At this point, the puberal growth spurt in girls is nearly complete. In boys, puberty begins later and lasts for nearly 5 years, in comparison to the $3\frac{1}{2}$-year period in girls. There are four stages of adolescence for boys. The first stage has to do with changes in the amount of fat in their body composition. Boys appear to be "chubby" and awkward in their physical appearance. Stage 2 begins about 1 year after stage 1 and is denoted by the beginning of the spurt in height and a decrease in the amount of body fat. Stage 3 is the peak velocity of height growth and occurs 1 year after stage 2. Facial hair appears on the upper lip, and there is a marked change in voice. Stage 4 begins 18 to 24 months after stage 3. The cessation of growth in height and the addition of facial hair on the chin mark the fourth stage of adolescence in boys.

Although orthodontists cannot necessarily modify growth (Wheeler et al. 2002, Tulloch et al. 2004), growth can affect treatment outcome. The principal goal in assessing physical growth status is to determine if the extent of facial growth remaining will have a positive or a negative effect on an individual's treatment. Modification of both hard- and soft-tissue–related dentofacial traits requires an understanding of the basic principles of craniofacial growth, development, and aging.

Dental History

There are two components of the patient's dental history. The first component is the patient's current commitment to maintaining oral health; that is, does the patient have a dentist, and what is the frequency of dental visits? The second component is the patient's actual dental history and the family history of dental or orthodontic conditions. A family history of variation in specific dentofacial traits is very important relative to future treatment planning. For example, in some families a strong chin may be a prized dentofacial trait. Treatment aimed at modifying this feature might be contraindicated based on family and patient preferences.

Perhaps the most important question for orthodontists in the dental history is, "Has the patient had any injuries to the face, mouth, or teeth?" Failure to record a traumatic injury to the teeth has potentially serious orthodontic consequences. There is a greater incidence of orthodontically induced root resorption in teeth with a history of trauma (Mirabella and Artun 1995, Andreasen et al. 2006). Lastly, the presence or absence of an oral habit in a child, an adolescent, or an adult will affect the potential outcome of orthodontic treatment (Ngan and Fields 1997).

Medical History

The importance of the medical history is to determine whether the patient has any pre-existing systemic conditions, which may affect orthodontic treatment. A survey of the medications the patient is taking will reveal possible systemic disease or metabolic issues. There are several classes of drugs that can affect orthodontic tooth movement (Tyrovola and Spryopoulos 2001) (Table 2.1).

For the most part, chronic medical conditions that are well controlled by medical treatment or drug therapy usually do not pose a greater risk for orthodontic complications. However, many endocrine disorders such as diabetes and thyroid disease are difficult to control and may pose a significant risk to the oral hard and soft tissues. If the orthodontist has any doubt about the patient's systemic health, a call to the primary care physician is appropriate. Occasionally, systemic disease will manifest itself in the oral cavity, and a referral to an oral medicine specialist is warranted.

The Doctor–Patient/Parent Interview

When the patient (and/or parent) presents to the orthodontic office for the initial examination, the orthodontist should have already gained a significant amount of insight into the patient's state of wellness via the health questionnaire. The goal of the patient/parent interview is to clarify and expand upon those data. The orthodontist must initiate a dialogue that will establish the patient's chief concern(s), motivation for seeking treatment, and expectation of treatment (Fig. 2.3).

Through a series of questions, the orthodontist should be able to ascertain why the patient is seeking his or her advice and what the patient's expectations of treatment are. If the patient is accompanied by his or her parent(s), then both parties should be asked these questions in order to determine whether the motivation for treatment is internal (from the patient) or external (from the parent, peers, or dentist). Armed with the data from the health questionnaire and the patient interview, the orthodontist can perform a more focused clinical examination of the patient's dentofacial complex.

Patient Autonomy

The center of debate regarding decision-making in orthodontics is whether the orthodontist or the patient should make the ultimate decision as to whether treatment is needed. In effect, this clash is between the concepts of paternalism and autonomy. *Paternalism* is "an action taken by one person in the best interest of another person without their consent" (Ackerman 1991). *Autonomy* is "a belief in the merit of individual self-determination" (Ackerman 1991). It has been suggested that autonomy be measured along four axes (Kukafka 1989). The first axis is "free action," whereby an individual acts free of coercion (internal or external). The second axis states that all actions are grounded in "rational deliberation," which refers to a logical consideration of

Table 2.1 Drugs that may affect orthodontic tooth movement.

Drug Class	Potential Effect on Tooth Movement
Bisphosphonates (e.g., alendronate)	Inhibition of tooth movement
Nonsteroidal anti-inflammatory drugs (NSAIDs) (e.g., indomethacin)	Inhibition of tooth movement
Corticosteriods (e.g., prednisone)	Acceleration of tooth movement
Thyroid hormone (e.g., levothyroxine sodium)	Acceleration of tooth movement

THE DOCTOR-PATIENT INTERVIEW

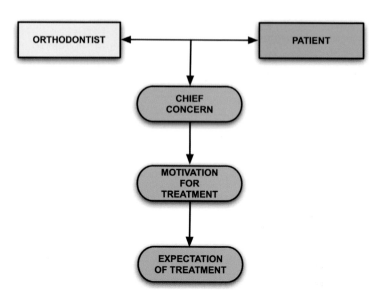

Figure 2.3 The key components of the doctor–patient interview.

fact. The third axis explains that actions must be "authentic"; they must be consistent with the person taking action. Last, the fourth axis discusses the degree of "moral reflection" behind an action, which represents how the actor applied his or her attitudes, values, and life plans to the action.

The conflict between autonomy and paternalism in orthodontist–patient communication arises relative to the amount of informative disclosure to the patient. If the orthodontist fails to disclose certain facts regarding a treatment decision, then the doctor is acting paternalistically and counter to the second axis of autonomy. The patient cannot rationally deliberate if he or she is denied any of the facts. Hence, patient autonomy is essential for acquiring informed consent.

Informed consent is "a social policy based on ethical guidelines and supported by legal precedence" (Ackerman 1991). It enhances the orthodontist–patient relationship through better communication. The following issues need to be discussed with the patient before seeking informed consent (Chiccone 1990):

1. A diagnosis must be presented in language that is easily understood by the patient.
2. A treatment plan explaining what procedures are recommended and how they will be performed must be presented to the patient.
3. Reasonable alternatives to the proposed treatment plan must be presented to the patient.
4. The probable sequelae of electing no treatment must be presented to the patient.
5. The potential risks, consequences, and possibility of secondary treatment must be presented to the patient.
6. The predicted outcome of treatment including the benefit to the patient and the probability of success must be presented to the patient.

The orthodontist must also understand three provisos before obtaining informed consent (Chiccone 1990). They are as follows:

1. The greater the potential injury, even if the risk is minimal, the greater is the obligation to inform the patient (e.g., risk of maxillary necrosis after Le Fort I surgery).
2. The greater the chance of a risk occurring even if the injury would be minimal, the greater is the obligation to inform the patient (e.g., risk of root resorption).
3. The more elective the proposed treatment, the more invasive the bodily intrusion will be considered in the event of an injury—thus, the greater the obligation to inform the patient (e.g., genioplasty for appearance reasons only).

One of the most important features of informed consent is describing to the patient the consequence of no treatment. At present, there is little scientific evidence regarding the adverse effects of an untreated variation in a dentofacial trait or traits. It is therefore important to explain to the patient that the prevailing concept of "normal" occlusion is based on conventional wisdom in dentistry and is supported by only anecdotal data. The long-term efficacy of orthodontic treatment—the net benefit and risks of intervention—is not fully understood (Vig 1991).

The Doctor—Patient/Parent Conference

After the orthodontist has the opportunity to clinically examine the patient, perform the appropriate diagnostic imaging, classify the patient's orthodontic condition(s), and develop treatment alternatives, he or she will meet with the patient (and/or parent) to discuss the findings and recommendations. The conference is divided into three components (Ackerman and Proffit 1995) (Fig. 2.4).

In the first component, the orthodontist details the patient's composite of dentofacial traits, reviews the list of orthodontic conditions encompassing the patient's chief concern, and presents possible treatment alternatives directed at resolving the patient's

THE DOCTOR-PATIENT CONFERENCE

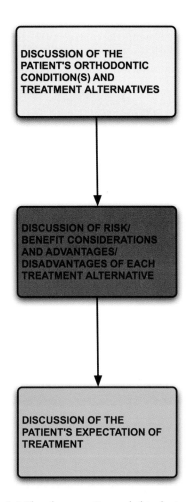

Figure 2.4 The three portions of the doctor–patient conference.

orthodontic condition(s). The second portion of the conference is a discussion of the risks and benefits of treatment and the advantages and disadvantages of the various treatment alternatives, including the option of no treatment. Patients and parents are often quite surprised to learn that there are multiple treatment options to select from. The third component of the conference is a discussion of the patient's expectations from treatment.

At the end of this dialogue, the orthodontist may state that treatment is being offered on an informed basis and may ask the patient to acknowledge that he or she understands there are risks as well as benefits pertaining to the treatment alternative that the patient selects. Although a "one-step" approach to initial examination, consultation, and initia-

tion of treatment has become very popular in orthodontics today, it is difficult, if not impossible, for an orthodontist to fulfill ethical responsibilities to the patient in this kind of practice management scheme.

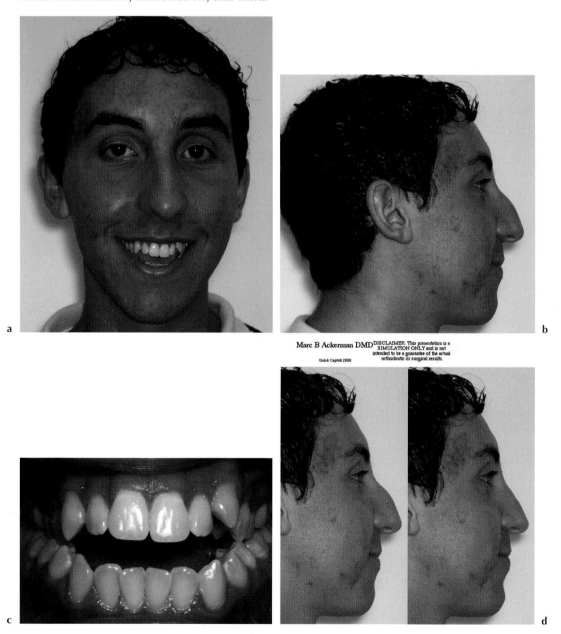

Figure 2.5 (**A–C**) Computer imaging software facilitates dialogue between the doctor and patient. This patient's chief concern was related to nasal form, chin projection, and the anterior open bite. (**D**) The treatment alternative of orthodontics, orthognathic surgery, and rhinoplasty was simulated using the morphing feature in Quick Ceph 2000 (Quick Ceph Systems, San Diego, California).

Enhancing Communication with Computer Software

Computer imaging software greatly enhances the patient's ability to visualize potential appearance changes resulting from orthodontics, orthognathic surgery, and plastic surgery (Fig. 2.5).

With the aid of morphing technology, an orthodontist can simulate the proposed changes in facial appearance for various treatment alternatives. By seeing the extent of facial change related to orthodontics alone or perhaps orthodontics in combination with orthognathic or plastic surgery, the patient is better equipped to make an informed decision about the treatment best suited to his or her needs.

Computer software that educates the patient about various orthodontic conditions and their treatment is also a very useful tool in doctor–patient communication (Fig. 2.6).

The orthodontist in either the initial examination or patient/parent conference can use on-screen digital images or videos to describe the patient's orthodontic condition and suggest appropriate treatment alternatives. Patients often have many questions regarding appliance design, application, and use. These types of software programs are exceedingly informative and easy to use.

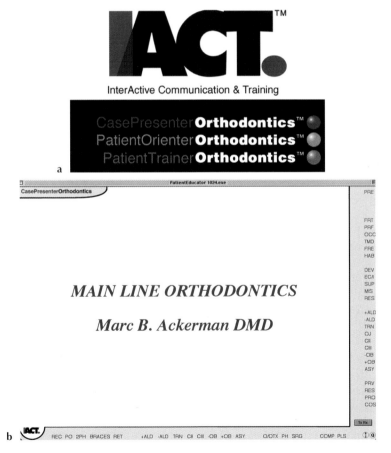

Figure 2.6 (**A–C**) Computer software that educates the patient about various orthodontic conditions and their treatment is a very useful tool in doctor–patient communication. (Images courtesy of InterActive Communication & Training-IACT, Birmingham, Alabama.)

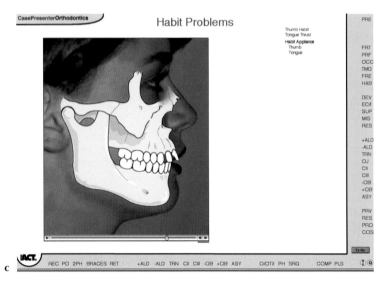

Figure 2.6 *Continued*

Communication During and After Orthodontic Treatment

Open lines of communication between the orthodontist and patient (or parent) are essential during and after active orthodontic treatment. In many cases, the orthodontist may need to make a mid-course correction, or there might be an unforeseen change in the patient's dental health status during treatment. A good policy is to apprise the patient of the progress at each visit and perhaps schedule a brief progress consultation with the patient at key stages of treatment. Chart notes should document the patient's level of compliance and ability to maintain oral hygiene. Problems in these two areas should be discussed with the patient or parents and followed up with a letter or e-mail with a copy to the patient's dentist discussing the risks of such behavior (Fig. 2.7).

The orthodontist cannot assume that a patient will remember all of the information that was presented at the pretreatment conference, and it will have to be reinforced throughout treatment.

When the patient is about to complete active treatment, it is crucial to explain the sequence of events comprising appliance removal and retention. The average orthodontic patient has forgotten that once active treatment ends, he or she must return to the orthodontist for follow-up visits. A good technique for encouraging patients to comply with the retention scheme is to show them their pretreatment and post-treatment images, highlighting which dentofacial traits were modified and how those traits may be prone to relapse or change in the future. Patients are routinely told that maintenance of tooth position will require indefinite (potentially lifetime) retainer wear. Time spent with the patient at the end of treatment will prevent the majority of misunderstandings and failures in compliance with retention. Successful communication in orthodontics is dependent on the orthodontist's ability to sustain an open dialogue with the patient throughout treatment and to *listen* attentively to the patient's questions, complaints, and needs.

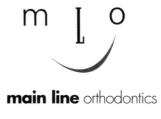

main line orthodontics

Marc Bernard Ackerman, D.M.D.
Diplomate, American Board of Orthodontics

Mr. & Mrs. James Edward Doe
1234 Main Street
Anywhere, USA 11211

RE: Jimmy Ed's Oral Hygiene and Appliance Care

Dear Mr. & Mrs. Doe,

As you may remember from our consultation appointment, keeping teeth and appliances clean is critically important during orthodontic treatment if we wish to finish with healthy gums and teeth. In Jimmy Ed's case, the teeth and gums show signs that improvement is needed in oral hygiene. We have carefully explained to Jimmy Ed how to brush correctly to get the teeth clean. In addition, I advise using Prevident toothpaste twice a day. I also recommend that Jimmy Ed see his dentist every four months during orthodontic treatment. Hopefully, this situation will improve soon.

Also, as mentioned during our consultation appointment, successful orthodontic treatment depends upon the patient exercising reasonable care in avoiding hard or chewy foods to prevent damage to the appliances. Damaged appliances need time to repair, but more importantly, they lengthen the time that will be required to complete treatment. More than an average amount of damage has occurred to the braces, and I am concerned that we are falling behind in our treatment schedule due to this problem.

Only if we are successful in solving these problems can treatment be completed in a reasonable amount of time.

Please call if you have any questions, and thanks, in advance, for your help.

Sincerely,

Marc B. Ackerman, D.M.D.

MBA/amk

cc: Dr. Joe Smith

931 Haverford Road • Bryn Mawr, Pennsylvania 19010-3819 • Office: 610-527-3678 • Fax: 610-527-6624
ackersmile@aol.com
Member American Association of Orthodontists

Figure 2.7 A library of form letters can be created using most orthodontic practice management software. This letter informs a patient's parents about a lapse in oral hygiene and repeated breakage of appliances.

REFERENCES

Ackerman, J.L. 1991. Autonomy versus paternalism in the decision making process: The doctrine of informed consent. In *Orthodontics at crossroads*, edited by J.G. Ghafari and C.F.A. Moorrees, pp. 49–60. Boston: Harvard Society for the Advancement of Orthodontics.

Ackerman, J.L., Proffit, W.R. 1995. Communication in orthodontic treatment planning: Bioethical and informed consent issues. *Angle Orthod* 65:253–262.

Andreasen, J.O., Bakland, L.K., Andreasen, F.M. 2006. Traumatic intrusion of the permanent teeth. Part 3. A clinical study of the effect of treatment variables such as treatment delay, method of repositioning, type of splint, length of splinting, and antibiotic on 140 teeth. *Dent Traumatol* 22:99–111.

Chiccone, M.U. 1990. Informed consent. *Perspective. The Dental RX* (publication of the Mid-Atlantic Medical Insurance Company) 3(2).

Kukafka, A.L. 1989. Informed consent in law and medicine: Autonomy v. paternalism. *J Law Ethics Dent* 2:132–142.

Marshall, W.A., Tanner, J.M. 1986. Puberty. In: *Human growth*, Vol. 2, Ed. 2, edited by F. Falkner and J.M. Tanner. New York: Plenum Publishing.

Mirabella, A.D., Artun, J. 1995. Risk factors for apical root resorption of maxillary anterior teeth in adult orthodontic patients. *Am J Orthod Dentofac Orthop* 108:48–55.

Ngan, P., Fields, H. 1997. Open bite: A review of etiology and management. *Pediatr Dent* 19:91–98.

Tulloch, J.F.C., Proffit, W.R., Phillips, C. 2004. Outcomes in a 2-phase randomized clinical trial of early class II treatment. *Am J Orthod Dentofac Orthop* 125:657–667.

Tyrovola, J.B., Spryopoulos, M.N. 2001. Effect of drugs and systemic factors on orthodontic treatment. *Quintessence Int* 32:365–371.

Vig, P.S. 1991. Orthodontic controversies: Their origins, consequences, and resolution. In: *Current Controversies in Orthodontics*, edited by B. Melson. Chicago: Quintessence Publishing Company.

Wheeler, T.T., McGorray, S.P., Dolce, C., Taylor, M.G., King, G.J. 2002. Effectiveness of early treatment of Class II malocclusion. *Am J Orthod Dentofac Orthop* 121:9–17.

Practice II

Clinical Examination of Dentofacial Traits

3

In contemporary orthodontic practice, the most critical step en route to enhancement of dentofacial traits is the clinical examination of the patient. Data acquired from this exercise form the basis for diagnosis and treatment planning. It is essential that adequate time be allotted for a thorough examination of the patient's dentofacial appearance and oral function in vivo. Although diagnostic imaging is a valuable complement to the clinical examination, it is not a substitute for direct hands-on assessment of the patient's dentofacial complex. As a starting point, the patient's chief concern will provide some insight into his or her perceived orthodontic need and guide the clinical examination. However, the chief concern should not limit the scope of the clinical examination. The three echelons of clinical appraisal of dentofacial appearance are *global*, *regional*, and *local* (Fig. 3.1).

The goal of this chapter is to describe a systematic method for the clinical examination of dentofacial appearance.

Self-perception and Observer-Perception of Facial Appearance in a Social Context

An individual's awareness of his or her facial appearance is derived largely by what they see in the mirror. We are all influenced, to a greater or lesser extent, by prevailing societal preferences for facial attractiveness. Thus, our image of self is in some measure a comparison of our own appearance compared to some tacit standard. Although self-image can be distorted (either positively or negatively), most would agree that our self-esteem can be very closely tied to our perception of our own relative attractiveness. Because most meaningful social interactions involve face-to-face contact, is it any wonder that most of us spend an inordinate amount of time in front of the bathroom mirror tending to facial blemishes and preening our hair in an attempt to enhance facial appearance? This self-assessment of facial appearance, which is limited in perspective by one's visual

CLINICAL APPRAISAL OF DENTOFACIAL APPEARANCE

GLOBAL

REGIONAL

LOCAL

SELF-PERCEPTION AND OBSERVER-PERCEPTION

Figure 3.1 The three echelons of clinical appraisal of dentofacial appearance. When performing a clinical examination, the clinician must ascertain which dentofacial traits are positively or negatively influencing the self-perception and the observer-perception of the patient.

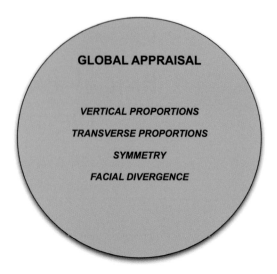

Figure 3.2 The elements of global appraisal of dentofacial appearance.

axis and peripheral vision, can be termed *self-perception*. It shapes an individual's appearance concept and influences his or her capacity for social engagement. Others, however, assess our facial appearance in multiple perspectives. This assessment of another's facial appearance can be called *observer-perception*. This feedback also to some extent shapes an individual's appearance concept and affects his or her capacity for social engagement through social cues. When performing a clinical examination, the orthodontist must ascertain which dentofacial traits are positively or negatively influencing the self-perception and the observer-perception of the patient.

Global Appraisal (Fig. 3.2)

Vertical Proportions

With self-perception and observer-perception in mind, clinical examination begins

with the global assessment of the full face oriented in natural head position (see Chapter 4). The patient should be evaluated both at rest and in dynamic motion (i.e., speaking and smiling). Faces can be broadly categorized as mesocephalic, brachycephalic, or dolichocephalic (Fig. 3.3).

The differentiation between these facial types relates to the proportionality of facial breadth to facial height, with brachycephalic faces being broader and shorter in comparison to the longer and narrower dolichocephalic faces. In general, the most attractive faces tend to be proportionate. Clinical examination begins with an appraisal of vertical proportionality. The face is vertically divided into equal thirds by horizontal lines adjacent to the hairline, the eyebrows, the nasal base, and the base of the chin (Fig. 3.4).

In the well-proportioned lower facial third, the upper lip makes up the upper third, and the lower lip and chin compose the lower two-thirds (Fig. 3.5).

Disproportion of the vertical facial thirds may be a result of many dental and skeletal factors, and these proportional relationships

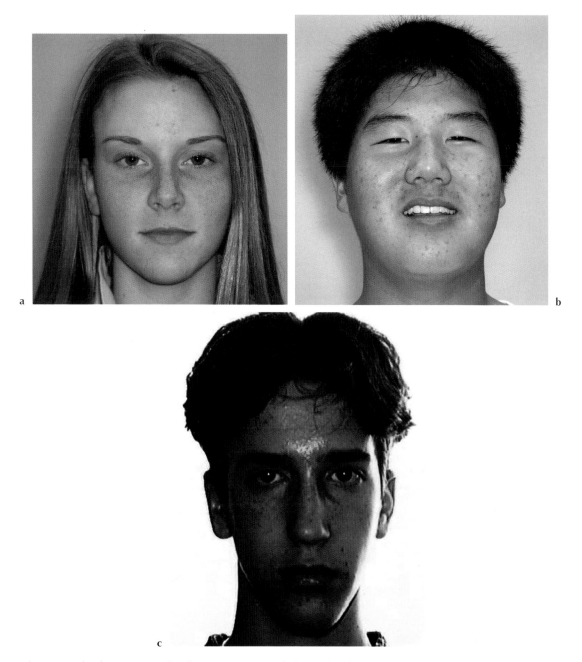

Figure 3.3 The three common facial types: (**A**) mesocephalic, (**B**) brachycephalic, and (**C**) dolichocephalic.

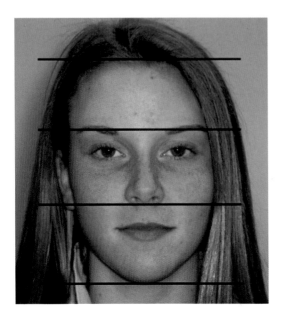

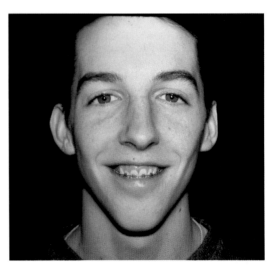

Figure 3.4 The proportionate face is vertically divided into equal thirds by horizontal lines adjacent to the hairline, the eyebrows, the nasal base, and the base of the chin.

Figure 3.6 The etiology of long lower facial height is related to either (1) vertical maxillary excess (VME) or (2) excessive chin height. The dentofacial traits that may be associated with VME are gummy smile, open bite, lip incompetence, and a steep mandibular plane as evidenced by gonial angle form. This patient has both VME and excessive chin height.

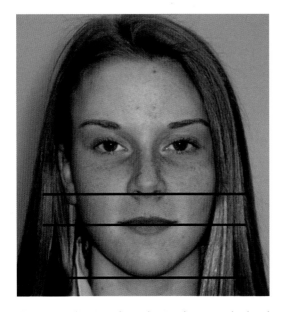

Figure 3.5 The upper lip makes up the upper third and the lower lip and chin compose the lower two-thirds of the lower facial third in the proportionate face.

may help define the contributing factors related to variation in dentofacial traits at the global level.

Discrepancies in Vertical Proportions

The etiology of a long lower facial height is related to vertical maxillary excess (VME) or excessive chin height. The dentofacial traits that may be associated with VME are gummy smile, open bite, lip incompetence, and steep mandibular plane with accentuated gonial angle form. Excessive chin height is measured from lower lip vermilion to the base of the soft tissue chin. The clinical features associated with excessive chin height are disproportion in the one-third upper lip–to–two-thirds lower lip/chin ratio (Fig. 3.6).

Differential diagnosis for a short lower facial height includes (1) vertical maxillary deficiency (VMD), (2) diminished chin height, or (3) posterior dental collapse sec-

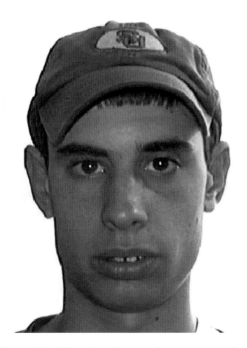

Figure 3.7 Differential diagnosis for short lower facial height includes (1) vertical maxillary deficiency, (2) diminished chin height, or (3) posterior dental collapse secondary to the loss of posterior dental support. This patient has a diminished chin height as well as an antero-posterior mandibular deficiency.

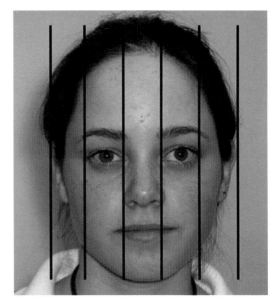

Figure 3.8 The assessment of facial breadth is best described by the rule of transverse fifths. The face is divided transversely into five equal parts from helix to helix of the outer ears. The five segments should be one eye distance in width.

ondary to the loss of posterior dental support. VMD is characterized by a short lower facial third, diminished maxillary incisor display at rest, and diminished incisor display on smile (Fig. 3.7).

Transverse Proportions

The assessment of facial breadth is best described by the rule of transverse fifths. The face is divided transversely into five equal parts from helix to helix of the outer ears (Fig. 3.8). The five segments should be one eye distance in width. Each transverse fifth should be individually examined and then assessed as a complete group.

The middle fifth of the face is delineated by the inner canthus of the eyes. The inner canthus of the eye is the inner corner of the eye containing the lacrimal duct. A vertical line from the inner canthus should be coincident with the lateral aspect of the alar base of the nose. Variation in this facial fifth could be due to transverse deficiencies or excesses in either the inner canthi or alar base. For example, hypertelorism in the syndromic craniofacial patient creates transverse disproportion. A vertical line dropped from the outer canthus and the inner canthus of the eyes frames the medial two fifths of the face. The vertical line at the outer canthus should be coincident with the gonial angles of the mandible. The outer two fifths of the face are measured from the outer canthus of the eye to the helix of the outer ear. Another significant frontal proportion is the midpupillary distance, which should be transversely aligned with the commissures of the mouth (Fig. 3.9).

Nasal anatomy in the transverse plane should also be assessed through proportionality. The width of the alar base should be approximately the same as the intercanthal

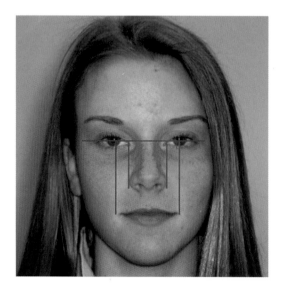

Figure 3.9 A vertical line from the inner canthus should be coincident with the lateral aspect of the alar base of the nose. Variation in this facial fifth could be due to transverse deficiencies or excesses in either the inner canthi or alar base. Another significant frontal proportion is the midpupillary distance, which should be transversely aligned with the commissures of the mouth.

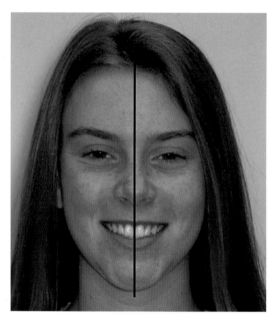

Figure 3.10 Facial symmetry is assessed relative to the midsagittal plane.

distance, which should be the same as the width of an eye. The width of the alar base is heavily influenced by inherited ethnic and racial characteristics.

Symmetry

Systematic examination of the patient's facial symmetry should be measured in the global appraisal. The assessment of facial symmetry is performed as follows.

Nasal Tip to Midsagittal Plane

The patient should elevate the head slightly and then, visualizing the nose in relation to the midsagittal plane, the orthodontist can view the position of the nasal tip. Any deviation of the nasal tip should be noted. The patient should be questioned as to any history of nasal trauma or nasal surgery for a deviated septum.

Maxillary Dental Midline to Midsagittal Plane

The maxillary dental midline should be recorded relative to the midsagittal plane (Fig. 3.10).

A discrepancy could be due to either dental factors or skeletal maxillary rotation, also known as *yaw* (see Chapter 4).

Mandibular Dental Midline to Midsymphysis

Standing behind the patient and viewing the lower arch from above is the best method to observe the mandibular dental midline relative to the midsymphysis (Fig. 3.11).

The patient should open the mouth for the orthodontist to view the lower arch and its relationship to the body of the mandible and symphysis. Lower dental midline discrepancies are usually a result of tooth-related issues such as dental crowding with shifted incisors, premature loss of primary teeth and subsequent space closure in preadolescents, congenitally missing teeth, or a unilaterally extracted tooth. If the lower dental midline

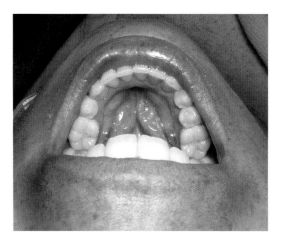

Figure 3.11 Standing behind the patient and viewing the lower arch from above is the best method to observe the mandibular dental midline relative to the midsymphysis.

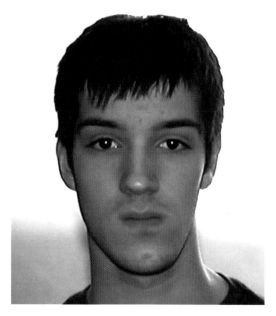

Figure 3.12 True mandibular asymmetry is suspected when, in closure from centric relation to maximum intercuspation, no lateral functional shift occurs. The asymmetric mandible may be due to an inherited asymmetric facial pattern or as a result of localized or systemic factors. This patient's true mandibular asymmetry is an inherited trait from his maternal side of the family.

is not coincident with the midsymphysis, it usually indicates a dental shift. However, chin asymmetry should also be considered.

Mandibular Asymmetry with or without Functional Shift

Mandibular asymmetry is suspected when the midsymphysis is not coincident with the midsagittal plane (Fig. 3.12).

An important diagnostic test is whether a functional shift of the mandible is present due to a skeletal or dental crossbite. Patients with bilateral crossbites will often shift their mandible to one side out of convenience when moving from centric relation to maximum intercuspation. This lateral shift signifies transverse maxillary deficiency rather than mandibular asymmetry. True mandibular asymmetry is suspected when, in closure from centric relation to maximum intercuspation, no lateral functional shift occurs. The asymmetric mandible may be due to an inherited asymmetric facial pattern or as a result of localized or systemic factors. A thorough history of traumatic injuries and a review of systems with the patient will help ascertain potential etiologies of mandibular asymmetry.

Chin Asymmetry

Facial asymmetry may be limited to the chin only. Measurement of the midsymphysis to the midsagittal plane is a good indicator of chin asymmetry, but the parasympheal heights should also be measured when chin asymmetry is suspected (Fig. 3.13).

The direct frontal view is recommended, but a view from the superior facial aspect (much like the evaluation of the mandibular dental midline) with the mouth closed also permits visualization of the chin to the body of the mandible and the midsymphysis.

Profile Analysis: Facial Divergence

Two aspects of the profile should be considered separately and then in combination. First, the convexity-concavity of the lips due to incisor position and the amount of lip support furnished by the dentition should be

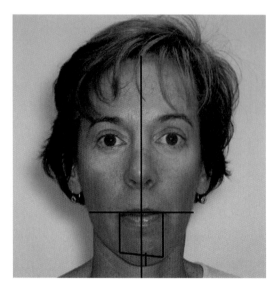

Figure 3.13 Chin asymmetry is assessed through measurement of the midsymphysis to the midsagittal plane as well as the parasymphyseal heights. This patient's left parasymphyseal height is longer than the right side.

fifths. The characterization of the nasal dorsum in profile view may indicate a dorsal excess or dorsal deficiency. The nasal tip is described as the most anterior point of the nose. The columella is the portion of the nose between the base of the nose and the nasal tip. It comprises the cartilaginous nasal septum and membranous septum. The nasolabial angle describes the inclination of the columella in relation to the upper lip. The nasolabial angle should be in the range of 90–120 degrees (Krugman 1981). The nasolabial angle is determined by several factors: (1) anteroposterior position of the maxilla, (2) anteroposterior position of the maxillary incisors, (3) vertical projection/vertical position of the nasal tip, and (4) soft-tissue thickness of the maxillary lip.

assessed. Second, the divergence anteriorly or posteriorly of the total facial profile, which reflects both the patient's head posture and global anatomic relationships, should be evaluated. The classic method for assessing the convexity of the face is to visualize a line from the soft tissue forehead to the anterior point on the upper lip to the soft tissue chin. This will form either a straight line (orthognathic face) or a concave or convex angle. A face in which the mandible is posteriorly placed is termed "posteriorly divergent." Conversely, a patient with mandibular prognathism would have an anteriorly placed mandible and is termed "anteriorly divergent" (Fig. 3.14).

Regional Appraisal (Fig. 3.15)

The Midface

Nasal form dominates the midface in frontal and profile views (Fig. 3.16).

As discussed above, nasal width should be proportionate according to the rule of facial

The Lower Face

The relative projections of the maxilla and mandible are assessed in the oblique (Fig. 3.17) and profile views.

The classic vertical facial thirds are also evaluated in profile view (Fig. 3.18).

The components of the lower face in profile are evaluated by (1) the relative degree of lip projection, (2) the labiomental sulcus, (3) the chin–neck length, and (4) the chin–neck angle. Lip projection is a function of maxillomandibular protrusion or retrusion, dental protrusion or retrusion, and/or lip thickness. The *labiomental sulcus* is defined as the fold of soft tissue between the lower lip and the chin and may vary greatly in form and depth. The clinical variables that can affect the labiomental sulcus are lower incisor position and vertical height of the lower facial third. Upright lower incisors and insufficient lower lip projection often result in a shallow labiomental sulcus. Conversely, excessive lower incisor proclination deepens the labiomental sulcus. Diminished lower facial height will often result in a deeper labiomental sulcus, whereas a patient with a long lower facial third has a tendency toward a flat labiomental sulcus. Chin projection is determined by

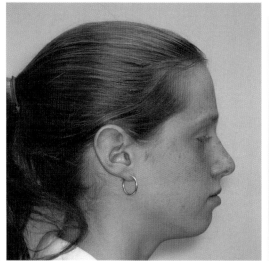
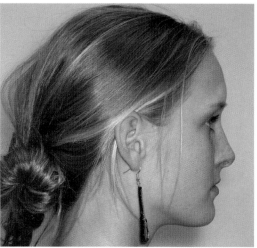

a

b

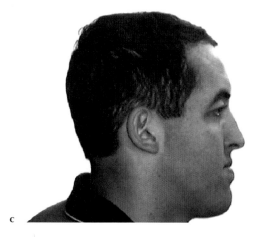

c

Figure 3.14 Convexity-concavity of the lips and anterior or posterior divergence of the profile interact to produce several profile combinations. The following examples demonstrate the spectrum of facial divergence: (**A**) a posteriorly divergent profile, (**B**) an orthognathic profile, and (**C**) an anteriorly divergent profile.

the amount of anteroposterior bony projection of the anteroinferior border of the mandible and the amount of soft tissue that overlays that bony projection. The angle between the lower lip, chin, and R point (the deepest point along the chin–neck contour) should be approximately 90 degrees. An obtuse angle often indicates (1) chin deficiency, (2) lower lip procumbency, (3) excessive submental adipose tissue, (4) retropositioned mandible, or (5) low hyoid bone. Another measure is the chin–neck length and chin–neck angle. The angle,

also termed the *cervicomental angle*, has been studied extensively in plastic surgery and orthognathic surgical literature (Sommerville et al. 1988) (Fig. 3.19).

A wide range of variation in neck morphology exists, and the cervicomental angle may vary between 105 and 120 degrees, with gender being a major consideration. The age of the patient should be considered with regard to this dentofacial trait. Soft-tissue "sag" in the cervicomental area is often due to the loss of skin elasticity and a function of aging. Excessive weight gain is another

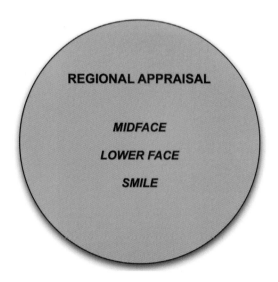

Figure 3.15 The elements of regional appraisal of dentofacial appearance.

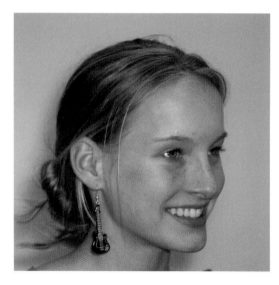

Figure 3.17 The relative projection of the maxilla and mandible are best visualized in the oblique view.

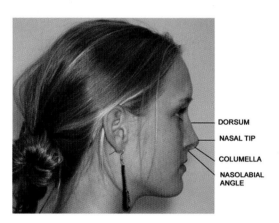

DORSUM
NASAL TIP
COLUMELLA
NASOLABIAL ANGLE

Figure 3.16 The components of nasal form.

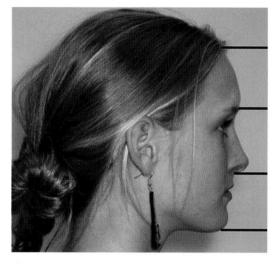

Figure 3.18 The classical vertical facial thirds are also evaluated in profile view.

important factor affecting the morphology of the chin–neck area.

The Smile

During clinical examination, it is important to differentiate between the two primary smile types—the social smile (posed) and the enjoyment smile (not posed) (Fig. 3.20).

The social smile is a *voluntary* smile developed by the patient, over time, in posing for photographs or in social settings. The enjoyment smile is an *involuntary* smile and represents the emotion one may be experiencing at that particular moment (e.g., laughing). In assessing smile dynamics, the social smile in most cases represents a repeatable smile (Rigsbee et al. 1988). It is important to note, however, that the maturation of the social smile occurs at different ages; therefore, the social smile in preadolescent patients may not be consistent over time. The range of variation in lip–tooth–gingival relationships during the social and enjoyment smiles should be assessed in the clinical examination.

Smile Style

The three styles of the dynamic social smile are (1) the commissure smile, (2) the canine smile, and (3) the complex smile (Rubin 1974). In the commissure smile, the corners

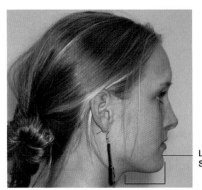

Figure 3.19 The components of the lower face in profile are evaluated by (1) the relative degree of lip projection, (2) the labiomental sulcus, (3) the chin–neck length, and (4) the chin–neck angle. The chin–neck angle may vary between 105 and 120 degrees, with gender being a major consideration.

of the mouth turn upward, followed by elevation of the upper lip due to the pull of the zygomaticus major muscles. In the canine smile, the upper lip is elevated uniformly without the corners of the mouth turning upward; that is, the entire lip rises like a window shade. In the complex smile, the upper lip moves superiorly as in the canine smile, but the lower lip also moves inferiorly in similar fashion.

Vertical Smile Traits

The vertical relationships between the incisal edges of the maxillary incisors relative to the lower lip and the relationship between the gingival margins of the maxillary incisors relative to the upper lip are important elements of the social smile. Optimally, the gingival margins of the maxillary canines should be coincident with the upper lip and the lateral incisors positioned slightly inferior to the adjacent teeth. In general, the gingival margins of the maxillary anterior teeth should be coincident with the upper lip in the social smile (Fig. 3.21). However, this is a function of the age of the patient, because children often show more teeth at rest and more gingival display on smile than do adults.

The following dentofacial traits related to the smile should be examined (Sarver and Ackerman 2005) (Fig. 3.22):

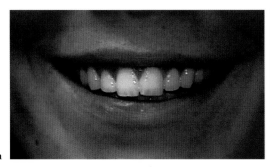
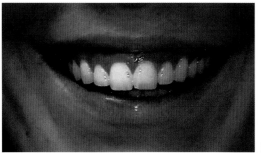

Figure 3.20 It is important to differentiate between the two primary smile types—the social smile (posed) and the enjoyment smile (unposed) during clinical examination. (**A**) The social smile is a *voluntary* smile developed by the patient, over time, in posing for photographs or in social settings. (**B**) The enjoyment smile is an *involuntary* smile, and represents the emotion one may be experiencing at that particular moment, such as laughing. Note the maximal lip elevation and excessive gingival display in this patient's enjoyment smile versus her social smile.

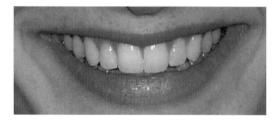

Figure 3.21 The vertical relationships between the incisal edges of the maxillary incisors relative to the lower lip as well as the relationship between the gingival margins of the maxillary incisors relative to the upper lip are important elements of the social smile.

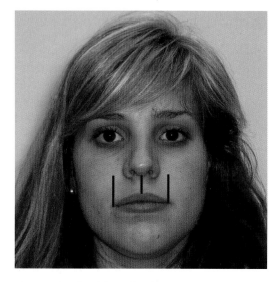

Figure 3.22 The philtrum height is measured in millimeters from the base of the nose at the midline to the most inferior portion of the upper lip on the vermilion. The commissure height is measured vertically from a line constructed at the alar base of the nose, to a parallel line passing through the commissures. Ideally, there should be no more than a 2- to 3-mm discrepancy between these two measures.

■ *Philtrum height.* The philtrum height is measured in millimeters from the base of the nose at the midline to the most inferior portion of the upper lip on the vermilion. The linear measurement of this trait is not as important as its relationship to maxillary incisor display and the height of the commissures of the mouth. In the adolescent, it is common to find the philtrum height less than the commissure height.

■ *Commissure height.* The commissure height is measured vertically from a line constructed at the alar base of the nose to a parallel line passing through the commissures.

■ *Interlabial gap.* The interlabial gap is the distance in millimeters between the upper and lower lips at rest or during smile.

■ *Amount of incisor shown at rest.* The amount of maxillary incisor shown at rest is an age-dependent dentofacial trait. One of the characteristics of aging is diminished maxillary incisor shown at rest and during smile.

■ *Amount of incisor display on smile.* When smiling, patients will either show their entire maxillary incisors or a percentage of those incisors. Measurement of the percentage of incisor display, when combined with the crown height measured next, aids the orthodontist's decision as to how much vertical tooth movement is required to attain the appropriate tooth display for the patient.

■ *Crown height.* The vertical height of the maxillary central incisors in the adult is measured in millimeters and is normally between 9 and 12 mm, with an average of 10.6 mm in males and 9.6 mm in females. The patient's age is a factor in measuring crown height because of the apical migration of the gingival tissues seen in adolescence.

■ *Gingival display.* The amount of gingival display on smile should be recorded. Natural aging will result in a diminution of this dentofacial trait. A mildly gummy smile is often judged more pleasing than a smile with insufficient tooth display. The following are possible etiologies contributing to excessive gingival display during smile:

1. Vertical maxillary excess (VME)
2. Short philtrum
3. Excessive upper lip animation
4. Short clinical crown height

■ *Smile arc.* The *smile arc* is defined as the relationship of the curvature of the incisal

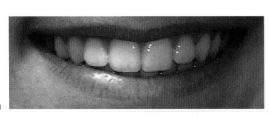
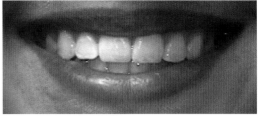

a   b

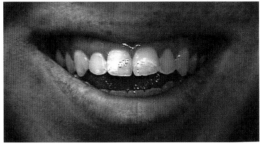

c

Figure 3.23 The smile arc is defined as the relationship of the curvature of the incisal edges of the maxillary teeth to the curvature of the lower lip in the posed social smile. (**A**) The consonant smile arc has the maxillary incisal edge curvature parallel to the curvature of the lower lip on smile. A flat (**B**) or reverse (**C**) smile arc is characterized by the maxillary incisal curvature being flatter or concave relative to the curvature of the lower lip on smile.

edges of the maxillary teeth to the curvature of the lower lip in the posed social smile (Ackerman et al. 1998). The consonant smile arc exhibits the maxillary incisal edge curvature parallel to the curvature of the lower lip on smile. A flat or reverse smile arc is characterized by the maxillary incisal curvature being flatter or concave relative to the curvature of the lower lip on smile (Fig. 3.23).

Transverse Smile Traits

Three interrelated factors affecting the appearance of transverse smile traits are arch form, buccal corridor, and the transverse cant or *roll* of the maxillary occlusal plane (see Chapter 4) (Fig. 3.24).

Arch form plays an important role in the appearance of the transverse smile dimension. In patients in whom the arch forms are narrow or collapsed, the smile may appear narrow and present inadequate tooth display transversely. An important consideration in widening a narrow arch form, particularly in the adult, is the axial inclination of the buccal segments. Patients whose posterior teeth are already flared laterally are not good candidates for dental expansion. Adolescent and adult patients, in whom the premolars and molars are upright, have greater capacity for transverse expansion. Orthodontic expansion and widening of a collapsed arch form can dramatically improve facial appearance and smile by increasing tooth mass projected laterally in the buccal corridors. Arch expansion can also have undesirable effects. Although a transverse increase in the dental arch may fill the buccal corridors, two undesirable side effects may result. First, full obliteration of the buccal corridor will create a "denture"-like smile. Second, when the anterior sweep of the maxillary arch is broadened, the smile arc is often flattened (Fig. 3.25).

Occasionally, clinical examination will reveal a transverse cant of the maxillary occlusal plane, also referred to as *roll* (see Chapter 4). A transverse cant of the maxilla can be due to (1) differential eruption and drift of the anterior and/or posterior teeth, (2) skeletal asymmetry of the mandible

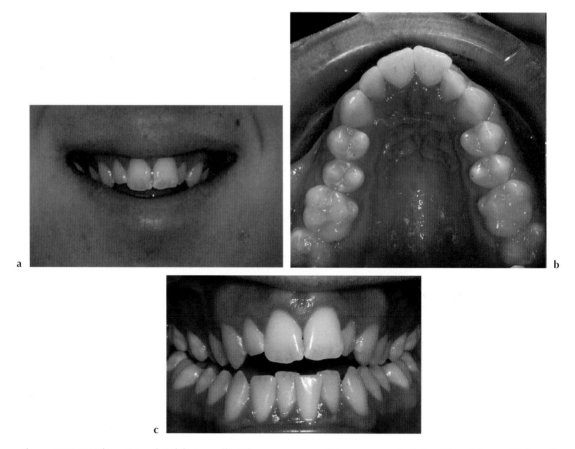

Figure 3.24 (**A**) Three interrelated factors affect the appearance of transverse smile traits: (1) arch form, (2) buccal corridor, and (3) the transverse cant or *roll* of the maxillary occlusal plane. (**B**) A saddle-shaped maxillary arch form is contributing to this patient's excessive buccal corridor in the social smile seen in **A**. (**C**) This intraoral view demonstrates the palatal inclination of the maxillary canines through the first permanent molars, which is negatively affecting arch form and buccal corridor.

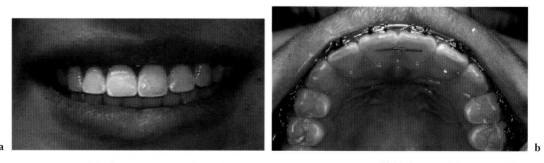

Figure 3.25 Arch expansion can have undesirable effects. Although a transverse increase in the dental arch may fill the buccal corridors, two undesirable side effects may result. (**A**) First, obliteration of the buccal corridor will create a "denture"-like smile. (**B**) Second, when the anterior sweep of the maxillary arch is broadened, the smile arc is often flattened.

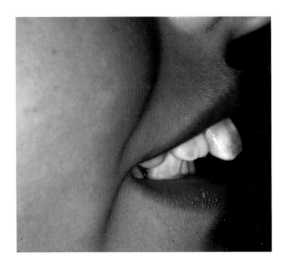

Figure 3.26 The anteroposterior dental traits that affect smile are overjet and incisor angulation. From an appearance standpoint, excessive overjet and flared incisors are two negatively connoted dentofacial traits.

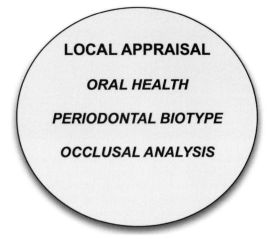

Figure 3.27 The elements of local appraisal of dentofacial appearance.

resulting in a compensatory cant to the maxilla, or (3) asymmetric vertical growth and development of the maxillary complex. Transverse smile asymmetry may also be due to soft-tissue considerations such as an asymmetric elevation of the upper lip.

Anteroposterior Smile Traits

Anteroposterior smile traits are described by the spatial orientation of the maxilla and maxillary teeth. In clinical examination, it is important to visualize the maxilla relative to the lower lip. The maxilla may be canted anteroposteriorly in a number of orientations. Deviations in maxillary orientation include a downward cant of the posterior maxilla, upward cant of the anterior maxilla, or variations of both. This maxillary rotation in the sagittal dimension is also referred to as *pitch* (see Chapter 4).

The anteroposterior dental traits that affect the smile are overjet and incisor angulation (Fig. 3.26).

From an appearance standpoint, excessive overjet and flared incisors are two negatively connoted dentofacial traits. When evaluated from an observer-perception standpoint,

individuals with excessive overjet and flared incisors are often labeled for these unflattering traits. However, when evaluated from a self-perception standpoint, an individual may not always perceive excessive overjet as a major detractor from his or her facial appearance in frontal mirror view. For example, some patients with skeletal Class II patterns have very pleasing smiles frontally but, when observed in profile view, show excessive overjet.

Local Appraisal (Fig. 3.27)

Oral Health

Local appraisal of dentofacial traits begins with an assessment of the patient's intraoral health. Clinical examination of the intraoral soft tissues should immediately reveal the patient's level of oral hygiene and general state of oral health. Inflammation in the gingival tissues and the extent of supragingival plaque/calculus should be noted. Periapical radiographs combined with a panoramic radiograph will reveal alveolar architecture and any evidence of horizontal or vertical bone loss. Suspected periodontal defects should be probed and the depths recorded.

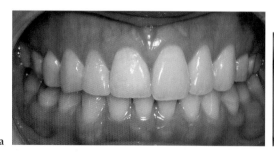
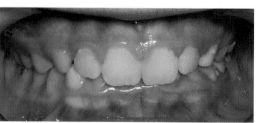

a   b

Figure 3.28 Periodontal biotypes. (**A**) The thin/scalloped biotype is characterized by the following: (1) a distinct disparity between the height of the gingival margin on the direct facial and that interproximally; (2) a delicate and friable soft tissue curtain; (3) the underlying osseous tissue scalloped with dehiscences and fenestrations often present; (4) a small amount of attached masticatory mucosa; (5) it reacts to insult via recession; (6) the contact areas of the adjacent teeth are located in the incisal or occlusal thirds; (7) triangular shaped teeth are present; (8) the contact areas of the adjacent teeth are small faciolingually and incisogingivally; and (9) steeper posterior cusps are present. (**B**) The thick/flat biotype is characterized by the following: (1) not as great a disparity between the height of the gingival margin on the direct facial and that interproximally; (2) a denser, more fibrotic soft tissue curtain; (3) a larger amount of attached masticatory mucosa; (4) the underlying osseous tissue is flatter and thicker; (5) it reacts to insult via increased pocket depth; (6) the contact areas of adjacent teeth are located more toward the apical; (7) square teeth are present; (8) the contact areas of the adjacent teeth are larger faciolingually and incisogingivally; and (9) flatter posterior cusps are present. (Modified from Weisgold and Starr 2004.)

The extent of attachment loss and degree of tooth mobility will influence tooth movement. In the presence of active disease, the teeth will move through the alveolus without concomitant remodeling. Tooth movement in a healthy periodontal apparatus will elicit alveolar remodeling. The buccal and labial mucosa should be examined for any pathology. Patients with recurrent aphthous ulcers will usually mention the most recent outbreak. Labial and lingual frenum attachments and their relationship to diastemata or gingival recession/clefting should be recorded. The clinical examination of the intraoral soft tissues should also include an assessment of the patient's swallow pattern, speech articulations, and tonicity of the lips and perioral musculature. Immature oral and pharyngeal function has a constellation of dentofacial traits associated with it, such as anterior open bite and flared incisors.

The occlusal grooves of posterior teeth should be checked with an explorer for any carious lesions. A patient's risk for future caries should be gauged relative to the present level of oral hygiene and the amount of existing dental restorations. Any decalcification,

enamel hypoplasia, or other tooth-related defects should also be recorded.

Periodontal Biotypes

As a structural unit, the dentogingival complex is defined by the relationship of the teeth to the alveolar bone and surrounding gingival tissues. The factors that influence the appearance of the dentogingival complex are the patient's periodontal status and past history of disease, the proximal and occlusal contacts of the teeth, the shape of the individual teeth, and the type of gingival architecture. The three periodontal biotypes are thick/flat, thin/scalloped, and pronounced thin/scalloped (Becker et al. 1997) (Fig. 3.28).

The *thin/scalloped biotype* is characterized by (Weisgold and Starr 2004):

1. Distinct disparity between the height of the gingival margin on the direct facial and that interproximally
2. Delicate and friable soft-tissue curtain
3. Underlying osseous tissue scalloped with dehiscences and fenestrations often present

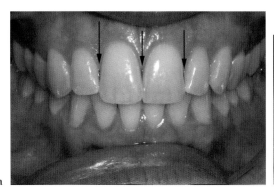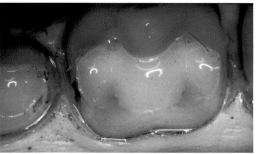

a   b

Figure 3.29 (**A**) After gingival recession has occurred in the thin/scalloped and pronounced thin/scalloped biotypes, "black triangles" are routinely seen in the anterior dentition. (**B**) A tissue section taken from a Mangabey monkey. The enamel of the tooth crowns was decalcified, showing the interdental tissue. Note the shape of the col. The anatomic features of the interproximal papillae are dependent on the morphology and position of the teeth. (Image courtesy of Dr. D. Walter Cohen.)

4. Small amount of attached masticatory mucosa
5. Reacts to insult via recession
6. Contact areas of the adjacent teeth located in the incisal or occlusal thirds
7. Triangular-shaped teeth present
8. Contact areas of the adjacent teeth are small faciolingually and incisogingivally
9. Steeper posterior cusps present

The *thick/flat biotype* is characterized by:

1. Not as great a disparity between the height of the gingival margin on the direct facial and that interproximally
2. Denser, more fibrotic soft-tissue curtain
3. Larger amount of attached masticatory mucosa
4. Underlying osseous tissue flatter and thicker
5. Reacts to insult via increased pocket depth
6. Contact areas of adjacent teeth located more toward the apical
7. Square teeth present
8. Contact areas of the adjacent teeth larger faciolingually and incisogingivally
9. Flatter posterior cusps present

Normally, the distance from the cementoenamel junction (CEJ) to the crest of bone on the direct facial in the healthy periodontium of a young adult is approximately 2 mm, with the gingival margin located on the enamel slightly incisal to the CEJ. In the pronounced thin/scalloped biotype, the distance between the CEJ and the bone on the direct facial is usually 3 to 4 mm. This results in the gingival margin being located at the CEJ or even on the root cementum.

In healthy oral cavities, the gingival papillae fill the space between the teeth 100% of the time when the distance from the contact point of the adjacent teeth to the interproximal crest of the bone is 5 mm or less. When the distance is 6 mm, the papillae do not fill the space completely in approximately 50% of patients, and when it is 7 mm or more, it does not fill the space in 75% of patients (Tarnow et al. 1992). After gingival recession has occurred in the thin/scalloped and pronounced thin/scalloped biotypes, "black triangles" are routinely seen in the anterior dentition (Fig. 3.29a).

Any interdental black triangles should be noted during clinical examination. The anatomy of the interdental tissue in the absence of an open contact and a state of gingival health is described as having two peaks connected interproximally in a triangular ridge depression. The shape of the interdental papilla when viewed from the

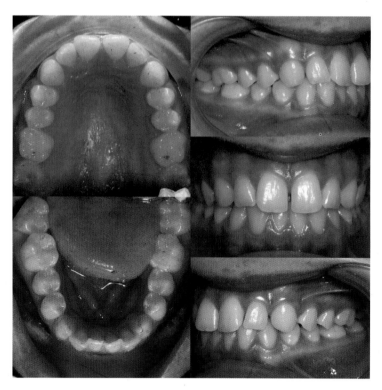

Figure 3.30 Intraarch and interarch relationships are described by the characteristics of dental alignment, crossbite (transverse dimension), Angle Classification (anteroposterior dimension), and bite depth (vertical dimension).

labial or lingual aspect is pyramidal. However, the inner portion of the papilla is triangle shaped as it encircles the proximal surfaces of the teeth, extending in a ridge-like depression connecting to the lingual aspect of the papilla. This interproximal shape has been termed the *col* (Cohen 1959, Fish 1961). The interproximal papilla, and more specifically the *col*, embraces the contact areas of adjacent teeth (Fig. 3.29b).

When diastemata are present, a saddle-type ridge is present. Thus, the anatomical features of the interproximal papillae are dependent on the morphology and position of the teeth (Goldman and Cohen 1966).

Occlusal Analysis (Fig. 3.30)

Clinically, the patient's occlusion should be examined both statically and dynamically.

The functional analysis should first establish the path of closure of the mandible and determine if the maximum intercuspal postion (centric occlusion) corresponds with the retruded contact position (centric relation). If there is a shift between these two positions, note any prematurities or convenience shifts that may exist. If there is a large anteroposterior discrepancy, the patient's occlusion should be classified in retruded contact position. If there is a small anteroposterior discrepancy, it is easier to classify the patient's occlusion in intercuspal position. Wear patterns on the cusps and incisal edges of teeth will reveal parafunctional movements of the jaws. Bruxism or clenching should be recorded. The temporomandibular joints and associated masticatory musculature should be palpated. Any crepitus or pain in the joints should be noted.

Intraarch and interarch relationships are described by the categories of dental alignment, crossbite (transverse dimension), Angle Classification (anteroposterior dimension), and bite depth (vertical dimension).

Dental Alignment

The maxillary and mandibular dental arches are described as either well aligned, crowded, or spaced. The extent of crowding or spacing is usually noted in millimeters. Individual teeth are described by virtue of their spatial position and degree of rotation. Therefore, an incisor could be described as severely rotated and in lingual version. The teeth present in the oral cavity should be counted. In the mixed dentition, a panoramic radiograph will aid the orthodontist in assessing whether the patient has the full complement of permanent teeth and the patient's dental age relative to chronologic age. The degree of root formation and calcification can be used to predict tooth emergence (Gron 1962). Any congenitally missing, lost, or supernumerary teeth should be noted. A description of teeth that have been severely worn or damaged due to trauma or parafunction should be recorded. Lastly, tooth size and shape should be evaluated. The proportions of tooth width–tooth height are evaluated beginning with the maxillary central incisors progressing posteriorly to the molars. Ideally, the maxillary central incisor's width should be in the range of 66% to 80% of its height (Gillen et al. 1994).

Crossbite (*Transverse Analysis*)

The assessment of transverse relationships is made initially from visual inspection of the arches intraorally. Posterior crossbites can present as either unilateral or bilateral discrepancies. The orthodontist must evaluate whether the crossbite is caused by a dental deviation or whether there is some skeletal component to the problem. To differentiate between dental and skeletal crossbites, the palatal configuration is examined. The palatal configuration is defined as high and constricted, average, or broad and flat. A high-constricted palate with a bilateral posterior crossbite usually indicates a maxillary transverse skeletal deficiency. As well, the orthodontist should evaluate the axial inclination of the buccal segments from the premolars moving posteriorly to the molars. Dental compensation for an underlying transverse discrepancy should be noted. Definitive diagnosis of transverse discrepancies will be accomplished through plaster or digital modeling of the dentition (see Chapter 4).

Angle Classification

In terms of static occlusion, the patient's Angle Classification should be noted. The Angle Class I relationship is such that the mesiobuccal cusp of the maxillary first permanent molar should rest in the buccal groove of the mandibular first permanent molar. The Angle Class II relationship exhibits a more anterior position of the mesiobuccal cusp of the maxillary first permanent molar, and the Angle Class III relationship exhibits a more posterior position of the mesiobuccal cusp of the maxillary first permanent molar. The degree of incisor overjet that accompanies any anteroposterior discrepancy should also be recorded.

Bite Depth

The vertical component of dental occlusion is bite depth. A patient's anterior bite depth is the amount of maxillary incisor overbite relative to the mandibular incisors. A patient can be described as having an anterior open bite, a satisfactory overbite, or an anterior deep bite. The posterior bite depth is usually characterized as being open, satisfactory, or collapsed. The latter is seen when the patient is missing unilateral or bilateral posterior dental units. Dental compensation in the vertical dimension relates to aberrations in the curve of Spee. The curve of Spee is measured by the arc extending from the cusp tips of the incisors posteriorly to the cusp tips of the first molar in sagittal view.

Integration of the Clinical Database

At the completion of the clinical examination, the orthodontist will have systematically examined the patient's dentofacial appearance and oral function at the global, regional, and local levels. The clinical database is now composed of two sets of information: (1) data acquired from the doctor–patient interview and (2) data acquired from direct clinical examination. At this point, the orthodontist should begin to integrate these two sources of clinical data. In many instances, a third set of data is required. This information is derived from a battery of patient-specific diagnostic imaging, which enables the orthodontist to visualize anatomic relationships not readily discernible on clinical examination.

REFERENCES

Ackerman, J.L., Ackerman, M.B, Brensinger, C.M., Landis, J.R. 1998. A morphometric analysis of the posed smile. *Clin Orthop Res* 1:2–11.

Becker, W., Ochsenbein, C., Tibbetts, L., Becker, B.E. 1997. Alveolar bone anatomic profiles as measured from dry skulls. Clinical ramifications. *J Clin Periodontol* 24:727–731.

Cohen, B. 1959. Morphological factors in the pathogenesis of periodontal disease. *Br Dent J* 107:31.

Fish, W. 1961. Etiology and prevention of periodontal breakdown. *Dental Progress* 1:234.

Gillen, R.J., Schwartz, R.S., Hilton, T.J., Evans, D.B. 1994. An analysis of selective tooth proportions. *Int J Prosthodont* 7:410–417.

Goldman, H.M., Cohen, D.W. 1966. Anatomy, histology, and physiology. In: *Introduction to Periodontia*, p. 3. St. Louis: C.V. Mosby Co.

Gron, A.M. 1962. Prediction of tooth emergence. *J Dent Res* 41:573–585.

Krugman, M.E. 1981. Photo analysis of the rhinoplasty patient. *J Ear Nose Throat* 60:56–59.

Rigsbee, O.H., Sperry, T.P., BeGole, E.A. 1988. The influence of facial animation on smile characteristics. *Int J Adult Orthod Orthognath Surg* 3:233–239.

Rubin, L.R. 1974. The anatomy of a smile: Its importance in the treatment of facial paralysis. *Plast Reconstr Surg* 53:384–387.

Sarver, D.M., Ackerman, M.B. 2005. Dynamic smile visualization and quantification and its impact on orthodontic diagnosis and treatment planning. In: *The art of the smile: Integrating prosthodontics, orthodontics, periodontics, dental technology, and plastic surgery in esthetic dental treatment*, edited by R. Romano, pp. 99–139. London: Quintessence Publishing Company, Ltd.

Sommerville, J.M., Sperry, T.P., BeGole, E.A. 1988. Morphology of the submental and neck region. *Int J Adult Orthod* 3:97–106.

Tarnow, D.P., Magner, A.W., Fletcher, P. 1992. The effect of the distance from the contact point to the crest of bone on the presence or absence of the interproximal dental papilla. *J Periodontol* 63: 935–996.

Weisgold, A.S., Starr, N.L. 2004. "Chapter 27: Restoration of the Periodontally Compromised Dentition." In: *Periodontics: Medicine, Surgery, and Implants*, edited by Louis F. Rose, Brian L. Mealey, Robert J. Genco, and D. Walter Cohen, pp. 677–678. St. Louis: Elsevier Mosby.

Imaging Dentofacial Traits

Diagnostic imaging of the dentofacial complex serves two important functions in clinical orthodontic practice. First, as was discussed in Chapter 2, imaging is a fantastic tool for enhancing communication between the doctor and the patient and/or the patient's parents. Second, imaging allows visualization of anatomic relationships that might not have been readily discernible during the clinical examination, further enhancing the orthodontist's ability to assess variation in dentofacial traits. Imaging can be categorized as either dynamic or static. Dynamic imaging is acquired from digital videography. Static imaging is obtained from stereo photogrammetry, conventional computed tomography (CT), cone-beam computed tomography (CBCT), and digital or plaster modeling of the dentition. The goal of this chapter is to discuss the latest and most advantageous imaging methods used in contemporary orthodontic practice and to explain how these tools assist the orthodontist in describing the spatial orientation of dentofacial traits.

Clinical Imaging Techniques

Dynamic Imaging

Digital Videography

Digital video and desktop computer software enable the orthodontist to record and view the idiosyncrasies of facial animation, such as speaking and smiling. The animated smile occurs at a faster rate than the human eye can process in real time. In fact, it often happens in less than a second (Ackerman 2003). Essentially, digital video records the equivalent of 30 still frames per second. A 5-second video clip of the patient will yield approximately 150 still frames for analysis. Thus, a very short video clip affords the orthodontist visualization of the range of lip–tooth relationships during speech and smiling.

Digital video should be taken in a standardized fashion with the camera at a fixed distance from the patient and the patient in natural head position (Fig. 4.1).

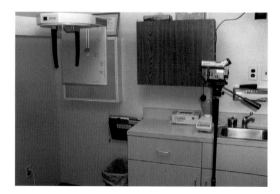

Figure 4.1 Digital video should be taken in a standardized fashion with the camera at a fixed distance from the patient and the patient in natural head position. In the author's practice, the digital video camera is mounted on a converted push-grip microphone stand. This set-up permits greater mobility than a traditional tripod. A built-in level positions the lens perpendicular to the true horizontal. The imaging studio uses ambient lighting; however, most digital video cameras give the user the option of attaching a supplemental light source.

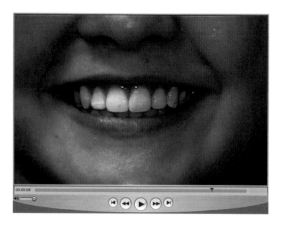

Figure 4.2 Digital video players allow slow motion assessment of the dynamic smile. This still frame of an unstrained posed social smile was acquired from Quick-Time Player Pro (Apple Computer, Inc., Cupertino, California).

Most digital video recorders have a viewfinder and a liquid crystal display (LCD) for viewing the subject while recording. The orthodontist should compose the smile in the LCD such that the base of the nose, the base of the chin, and several millimeters lateral to the commissures form the boundaries of the smile. At the present time, an ear-rod from a radiographic head holder is used to stabilize the patient's head, which eliminates any blurriness or chatter in the recording. Younger patients tend to bob their heads more than do adults when speaking. The patient is asked to say a short phrase and then asked to smile. Passive coaching encourages the patient to give a natural unstrained posed social smile followed by an enjoyment smile. The clinical assistant merely instructs the patient to "smile." Once the patient has given a natural unstrained posed social smile, the assistant will then ask for a "real big" smile in the hope of eliciting an enjoyment smile. The raw digital video is downloaded to the computer desktop, then compressed and saved in the .mov or .avi file type (Fig. 4.2). Digital video players allow slow motion assessment of the dynamic smile.

The orthodontist should review the video clip and select the smile frame that best represents the patient's natural unstrained posed social smile. Quantitative and qualitative analysis of lip–tooth–gingival relationships as described in Chapter 3 are easily accomplished with the aid of digital videography. As well, the orthodontist can review the video clip with the patient in order to familiarize the patient with his or her own smile. There are some preliminary data supporting the idea that clinicians can train their adult patients to give repeatable social smiles over time (Dong et al. 1999). However, there is questionable repeatability of posed social smiles in children. It has been postulated that adolescents undergo a maturational sequence in learning how to smile (Ackerman et al. 1998).

Static Imaging

Stereo Photogrammetry

Photogrammetry is defined as "the art, science, and technology of obtaining reliable information about physical objects and the environment through processes of recording, measuring, and interpreting photographic images and patterns of recorded radiant electromagnetic energy and other phenomena" (McGlone 2004). Photogrammetry can also be thought of as the sciences of geometry, mathematics, and physics that use the image of a three-dimensional scene on a two-dimensional piece of film to reconstruct a

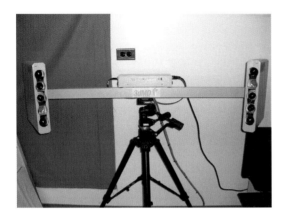

Figure 4.3 The 3dMD stereo photogrammetric scanner (3dMD, Atlanta, Georgia). It consists of an array of digital cameras used to perform surface imaging of the patient's face. A quick scan will generate a clinically accurate three-dimensional digital model of the patient's face.

reliable and accurate model of the original three-dimensional scene. Stereo photogrammetry is based on the concept of stereoviewing, which is rooted in the fact that humans naturally view their environment in three dimensions. Each eye sees a single scene from slightly different perspectives. The brain deciphers the difference, makes a computation, and then conveys the third dimension.

Applying the sophisticated principles of stereo photogrammetry, the orthodontist can use a commercially available array of digital cameras to perform surface imaging of the patient's face (Fig. 4.3).

A quick scan will generate a clinically accurate three-dimensional digital model of the patient's face (Fig. 4.4).

Proprietary software is used for image manipulation and volumetric measurement. By rotating the image along its vertical axis on the computer screen, the orthodontist can simulate how observers perceive a patient's facial appearance. The three-dimensional rendering of the patient's face enhances the orthodontist's ability to discuss global and regional variation in dentofacial traits during the doctor–patient conference.

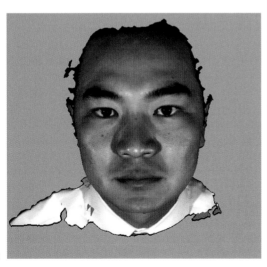
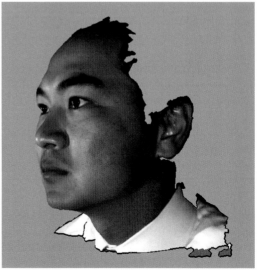

a   b

Figure 4.4 An actual 3dMD facial scan. (**A**) Frontal view. (**B**) Oblique view. (Images courtesy of Dr. Hideo Nakanishi, Department of Orthodontics, Temple University School of Dentistry, Philadelphia, Pennsylvania.)

Conventional Computed Tomography

CT is a method of patient imaging in which a thin x-ray beam rotates around the patient. Small detectors measure the amount of x-rays that pass through the particular area of interest. A computer analyzes the data to construct a cross-sectional image. These images can be stored, viewed on a monitor, or printed on film. In addition, stacking the individual images, or slices, can create three-dimensional models of patient anatomy. As the CT scanning takes place, the table will advance the horizontally lying patient at small intervals through the scanner. Modern spiral CT scanners can perform the examination in one continuous motion. Generally, complete scans will only take a few minutes. However, additional contrast-enhanced or higher-resolution scans will add to the scan time. The latest multidetector scanners can image an entire body, head to toe, in less than 30 seconds.

CT and three-dimensional imaging techniques are essential for assessing impacted teeth (Ericson and Kurol 1988, Chen et al. 2006). From a diagnosis and treatment-planning standpoint, the orthodontist must precisely establish the spatial position of an impacted tooth in relation to adjacent roots and other anatomical structures and then devise a mechanotherapy that avoids collateral damage. From a risk management standpoint, the clinician should know if there is any existing root resorption or pathology that has occurred due to the ectopically erupting or impacted tooth and then inform the patient of the risks associated with orthodontically assisting the eruption of that tooth (Fig. 4.5).

Conventional planar radiography is incapable of predictably detecting whether initial resorption has occurred on the palatal or labial aspect of roots adjacent to impacted teeth. Many therapeutic misadventures could be avoided by using CT imaging to guide surgical exposure and orthodontic movement of ectopic teeth.

Cone-Beam Computed Tomography

CBCT is specifically designed to image the hard tissues of the dentofacial complex. Conventional CT scanning is achieved through a helical fan-beam, providing thin-sliced images in the axial plane. The CBCT technique involves the patient seated in the scanner with the x-ray source and reciprocating detector synchronously moving around the patient's head in a single 360-degree scan (Fig. 4.6).

CBCT provides the orthodontist with a "real-time" image in the axial plane as well as two-dimensional images in the coronal, sagittal, and even oblique planes. This process is referred to as multiplanar reformation (Scarfe et al. 2006). CBCT data are also receptive to reformation in a volume, rather than a slice, which provides three-dimensional reconstructions (Fig. 4.7).

CBCT provides distinct images of highly contrasted anatomical structures and in particular is very useful for evaluating bone (Sukovic 2003) (Fig. 4.8).

The advantages of CBCT versus CT are (1) x-ray beam limitation (lower radiation dose) (Cohnen et al. 2002), (2) image accuracy (higher resolution due to isotropic voxels [equal in three dimensions]), (3) rapid scan time (averaging 10–70 seconds), (4) images that can be viewed immediately on the computer screen in a clinical office setting, (5) reduced image artifact (due to any metal in the oral cavity), and (6) lower cost. For these reasons, CBCT is rapidly supplanting conventional CT and conventional radiography in clinical orthodontic practice. The practice of routinely taking lateral radiographs of the skull is unwarranted. These two-dimensional plane films provide tremendously little insight into the three-dimensional spatial orientation of the hard-tissue components of the dentofacial complex.

Modeling the Dentition

Plaster models of the teeth, the traditional diagnostic record from the inception of

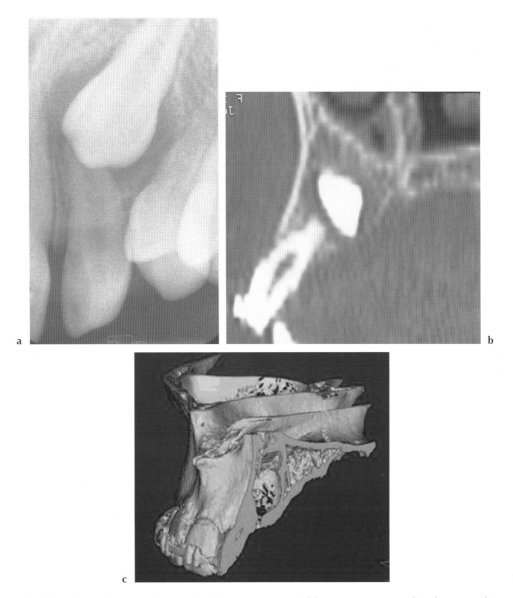

Figure 4.5 CT and three-dimensional imaging techniques are essential for assessing impacted teeth. From a diagnosis and treatment-planning standpoint, the orthodontist must precisely establish the spatial position of an impacted tooth in relation to adjacent roots and other anatomical structures and then devise a mechanotherapy that avoids collateral damage. (**A**) A periapical x-ray indicates that tooth No. 11 is ectopically erupting. The tooth was not palpable intraorally and other radiographs determined that it was palatally impacted. (**B**) A slice from a spiral CT scan clearly shows resorption of the root of tooth No. 10. (**C**) A three-dimensional reconstruction of the patient's maxilla, sectioned through the long axis of tooth No. 10. The crown of tooth No. 11 has been subtracted from the image showing the damage to the adjacent root of tooth No. 10.

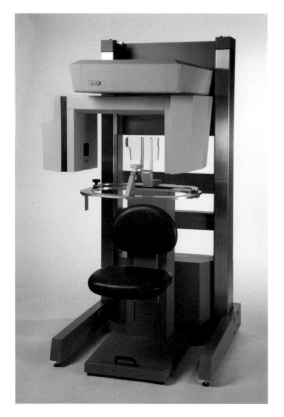

Figure 4.6 The i-CAT cone-beam computed tomography (CBCT) system. The CBCT technique involves the patient seated in the scanner with the x-ray source and reciprocating detector synchronously moving around the patient's head in a single 360-degree scan. (Image courtesy of Imaging Sciences International, Inc., Hatfield, Pennsylvania, and their public relations firm, Gregory FCA Communications, Ardmore, Pennsylvania).

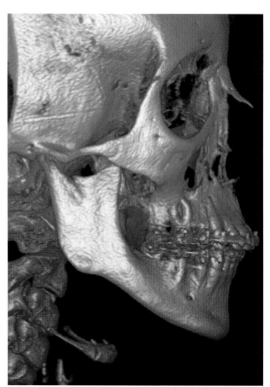

a

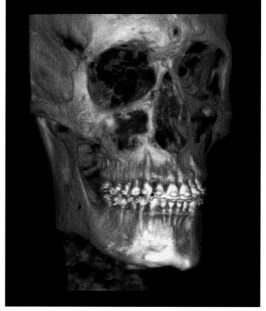

b

Figure 4.7 A three-dimensional image of the hard tissues of the dentofacial complex in (**A**) lateral and (**B**) oblique views, which were derived from an i-CAT CBCT scan using 3-DVR (three-dimensional volume-rendering software). (Images courtesy of Imaging Sciences International, Inc., Hatfield, Pennsylvania, and their public relations firm, Gregory FCA Communications, Ardmore, Pennsylvania).

orthodontics, have always been used to view the relationships of the teeth from any orientation (Fig. 4.9).

Currently, virtual models of the dentition viewed on a two-dimensional computer screen are replacing plaster models in clinical practice (Fig. 4.10).

Impressions are taken and then sent to a commercial facility for three-dimensional scanning. Virtual models are created, and the orthodontist can manipulate and measure

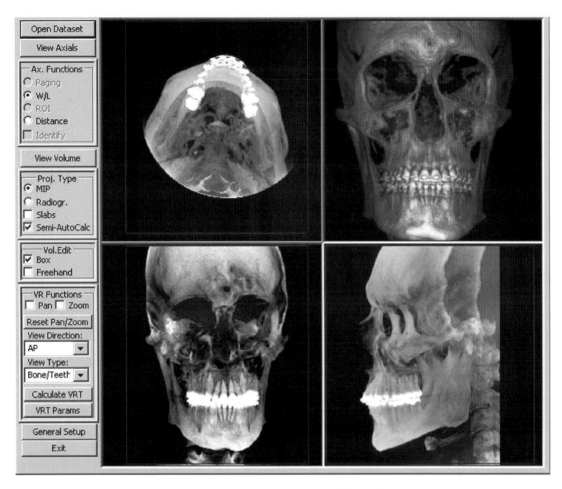

Figure 4.8 A collection of images taken from an i-CAT CBCT scan. The two lower images are maximum intensity projections (MIP). MIP is a thickening technique that displays only the highest voxel value within a particular thickness. It produces a "pseudo" three-dimensional structure and is excellent for depicting the surface morphology of the dental and skeletal hard tissues. (Images courtesy of Imaging Sciences International, Inc., Hatfield, Pennsylvania, and their public relations firm, Gregory FCA Communications, Ardmore, Pennsylvania).

them using proprietary software. In the future, a scan directly in the mouth will eliminate alginate impressions of the teeth in order to produce virtual models. Using a mouse, the orthodontist can rotate the on-screen virtual models, simulating three-dimensional plaster models.

The software technology for digital modeling is still in its infancy and has not fully replicated the diagnostic advantages of conventional plaster models. For instance, model surgery prior to fabrication of splints for orthognathic surgery still requires the use of plaster models. However, there are several orthodontic systems on the market that use digital modeling for appliance fabrication, wire construction, bracket placement, and prediction of tooth movement. The hope in the future is that digital modeling will facilitate the fabrication and application of highly efficient and effective custom-made orthodontic appliances.

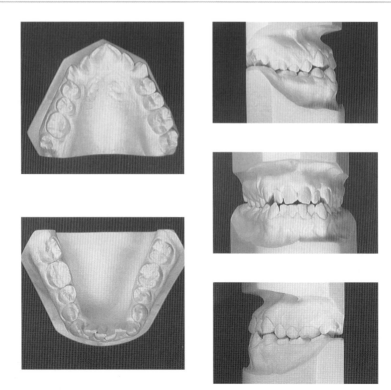

Figure 4.9 Plaster models of the teeth, the traditional diagnostic record from the inception of orthodontics, have always been used to view the relationships of the teeth from any orientation.

The Spatial Orientation of Dentofacial Traits

Pitch, Roll, and Yaw

The advent of CBCT and stereo photogrammetry makes it possible to directly view three-dimensional relationships within the dentofacial complex (Fig. 4.11).

Historically, orthodontic diagnosis addressed only three of the six characteristics required for describing the position of the teeth in the face and the orientation of the head. A total description of these relationships is analogous to what is required to describe the position of an airplane in space (Ackerman et al. 2007).

Three-dimensional movement in space is defined by translation (forward/backward, up/down, right/left) combined with rotation about three perpendicular axes (pitch, roll, and yaw) (Fig. 4.12). By adding these rotational axes into the characterization of dentofacial traits, the orthodontist has greater accuracy in description (Fig. 4.13).

Orientation of the Head and Lines of Occlusion

Although the importance of evaluating dentofacial traits in all three planes of space was emphasized during the clinical examination, the orientation of the head as well as of the teeth and jaws was not fully discussed. Natural head position (NHP) is the most rational physiologic and anatomic orientation for evaluating the face, jaws, and teeth (Moorees and Kean 1958). NHP is obtained by having the individual fix his or

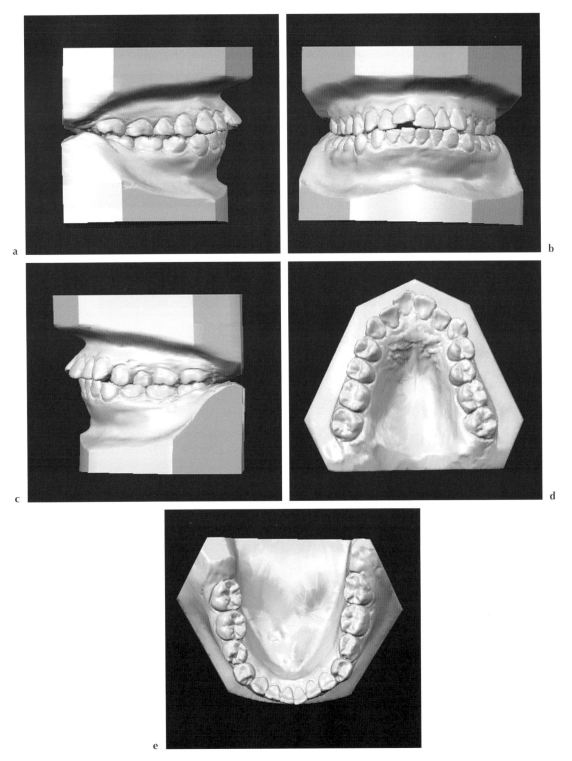

Figure 4.10 (**A–E**) Virtual models are created via a scan of alginate impressions. The orthodontist can manipulate and measure digital models using proprietary software. These images of digital models represent the traditional views used for occlusal analysis. (Images taken from a digital patient record created by OrthoCAD Digital Models, Cadent, Carlstadt, New Jersey.)

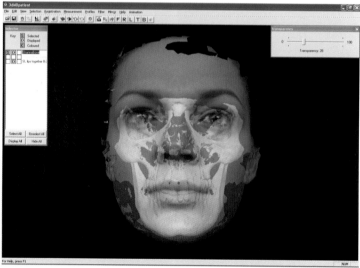

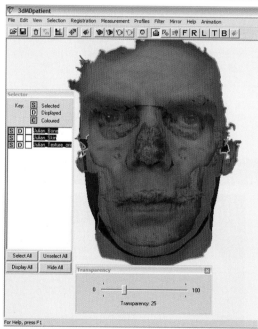

Figure 4.11 The advent of CBCT and stereo photogrammetry make it possible to directly view three-dimensional relationships within the dentofacial complex. (**A**) An integrated image using scans from the i-CAT CBCT system and the 3dMD system. (**B**) Proprietary software allows the clinician to adjust the transparency of the soft-tissue layers, which improves visualization of hard–soft tissue interrelationships. (Images Courtesy of Imaging Sciences International, Inc., Hatfield, Pennsylvania, and their public relations firm, Gregory FCA Communications, Ardmore, Pennsylvania)

her gaze at a distant object or at his or her own eyes in a wall-mounted mirror. Once the patient's visual axis is focused, the head will be oriented in NHP. Clinical examinations should be done with the head in NHP, imaging should be taken in NHP, and the orientation of three-dimensional images should be corrected to NHP. With the patient in NHP, the teeth and jaws can be oriented to the rest of the dentofacial complex using what is termed the *functional line of occlusion.*

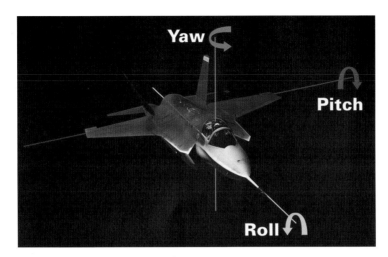

Figure 4.12 Three-dimensional movement in space is defined by translation (forward/backward, up/down, right/left) combined with rotation about three perpendicular axes (pitch, yaw, and roll). A complete description of a plane's orientation in space requires consideration of all six attributes. (Reprinted from Ackerman, J.L., Proffit, W.R., Sarver, D.M., Ackerman, M.B., Kean, M.R. Pitch, roll, and yaw: Describing the spatial orientation of dentofacial traits. *Am J Orthod Dentofacial Orthop* Vol. 131, 2007, with permission from the American Association of Orthodontists.)

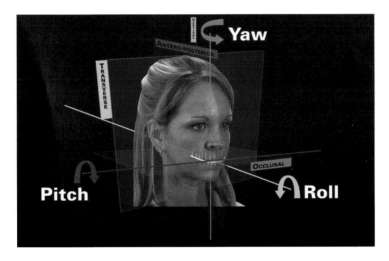

Figure 4.13 Three-dimensional analysis of the orientation of the head, jaws, and dentition is incomplete without also considering the three rotational axes of pitch, roll, and yaw in addition to the antero-posterior, transverse and vertical planes. (Reprinted from Ackerman, J.L., Proffit, W.R., Sarver, D.M., Ackerman, M.B., Kean, M.R. Pitch, roll, and yaw: Describing the spatial orientation of dentofacial traits. *Am J Orthod Dentofacial Orthop* Vol. 131, 2007, with permission from the American Association of Orthodontists.)

For more than a century, there has been a quest in orthodontics for a practical and reliable method of orienting the teeth to the jaws and face. It was postulated that if the buccal occlusal line of the mandibular dental arch was coincident with the line of the central fossae of the maxillary dental arch and if the teeth in the arches were well aligned, ideal occlusion would result (Angle 1899). These lines, referred to as the functional line of

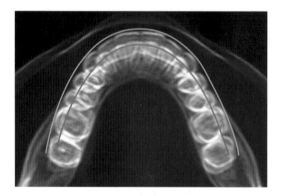

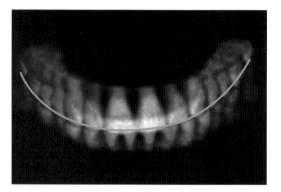

Figure 4.14 A submental-vertex CBCT view of an individual with normal occlusion. Angle's line of occlusion (red) runs along the buccal cusps and incisal edges of the mandibular teeth, and along the central fossae and cingulae of the maxillary teeth. Perfect alignment of the maxillary and mandibular lines is the condition for Angle's ideal occlusion. If a patient has an asymmetry characterized by rotation of the maxilla, mandible, dentition, or any of the above around the vertical axis, it can be detected in this radiographic projection. The second line (green), which follows the facial surfaces of the maxillary teeth, is the esthetic line of the dentition. It is valuable in evaluating lip–tooth relationships and the orientation of the dentition relative to pitch, roll, and yaw. (Image courtesy of Dolphin Imaging and Management Solutions, Chatsworth, California; reprinted from Ackerman, J.L., Proffit, W.R., Sarver, D.M., Ackerman, M.B., Kean, M.R. Pitch, roll, and yaw: Describing the spatial orientation of dentofacial traits. *Am J Orthod Dentofac Orthop* Vol. 131, 2007, with permission from the American Association of Orthodontists.)

Figure 4.15 A cross-sectional "block" of a CBCT image can be manipulated on the computer screen around all three rotational axes. This image is a different perspective of the same image shown in Figure 4.14. (Images courtesy of Dolphin Imaging and Management Solutions, Chatsworth, California; reprinted from Ackerman, J.L., Proffit, W.R., Sarver, D.M., Ackerman, M.B., Kean, M.R. Pitch, roll, and yaw: Describing the spatial orientation of dentofacial traits. *Am J Orthod Dentofac Orthop* Vol. 131, 2007, with permission from the American Association of Orthodontists.)

occlusion, are hidden from view when the maxillary and mandibular teeth contact. The functional line of occlusion describes the positions of the teeth within the dental arch and serves as a reference for assessing arch form, arch symmetry, and curve of Spee (Fig. 4.14).

There is a significant distinction between the occlusal plane and the functional line of occlusion. The occlusal plane is a flat two-dimensional construction, versus the line of occlusion, which is a three-dimensional structure created by the curve of Spee and lack of bilateral vertical symmetry. When the upper and lower lines of occlusion are misaligned, one cannot describe their relationship using planes.

The functional line of occlusion illustrates arch form, arch width, and symmetry. It does not describe the position of the anterior teeth relative to the facial soft tissues, that is, anterior tooth display and smile arc. In order to describe the dental and soft-tissue contributions to anterior tooth display, another line must be used. This line, the *esthetic line* of the dentition, follows the facial surfaces of the maxillary anterior and posterior teeth (Fig. 4.15).

The orientation of both the functional line of occlusion and the esthetic line of the dentition should be described using an *x*, *y*, *z* coordinate system in combination with pitch, roll, and yaw.

In this system, an excessive upward/downward rotation of the esthetic line of the dentition would be denoted as *pitch* (up or down, anteriorly or posteriorly). What is often referred to as a transverse cant of the occlusal plane, viewed relative to a skeletal reference plane like the interocular line or a soft-tissue reference plane like the intercommissure line, is described as *roll* of the esthetic line of the dentition and the func-

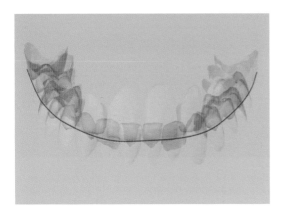

Figure 4.16 The advent of three-dimensional imaging enables the orthodontist to precisely visualize the orientation of the functional line of occlusion. An image similar to Figure 4.15 was extracted from digital models. The clinician is able to gain the same spatial information without the patient being exposed to x-ray radiation. (Images courtesy of OrthoCAD Digital Models, Cadent, Carlstadt, New Jersey; reprinted from Ackerman, J.L., Proffit, W.R., Sarver, D.M., Ackerman, M.B., Kean, M.R. Pitch, roll, and yaw: Describing the spatial orientation of dentofacial traits. *Am J Orthod Dentofac Orthop* Vol. 131, 2007, with permission from the American Association of Orthodontists.)

tional line of occlusion (up or down on one side or the other). Rotation of the functional line of occlusion and the esthetic line of the dentition to one side or the other, around a vertical axis, is described as *yaw*. The effect of *yaw* is visualized in dental and/or skeletal midline deviations, with a unilateral Angle Class II or Class III molar relationship. *Yaw* was omitted from previous classifications because it was difficult to detect during clinical examination and was rarely visible in conventional diagnostic imaging. The advent of three-dimensional imaging enables the orthodontist to precisely visualize the orientation of the functional line of occlusion (Fig. 4.16).

Clinical Practice Considerations

The orientations of both the line of occlusion and the esthetic line of the dentition are essential for diagnosis, treatment planning, and mechanotherapy. From a treatment standpoint, the orientation of the line of occlusion has far-reaching clinical significance (Burstone and Marcotte 2000). Interactions of the functional and esthetic lines are encountered routinely in the effect of interarch elastics, which tend to tip the line of occlusion up or down in either the anterior or posterior regions of the arch.

The orientation of the functional line of occlusion and esthetic line of the dentition affect anterior tooth display during speech and smiling. The *pitch* and *level* of the functional line of occlusion are both important determinants of treatment for undesirable anterior tooth display. For example, the anterior teeth could be pitched too far down, or the whole maxillary dentoalveolar complex could be positioned too far up or down although its *pitch* is normal. The intercommissure line (Morley and Eubank 2001) is a useful reference line for evaluating *pitch* and its effect on anterior tooth display and lip–tooth relationships. Patients with an anterior open bite often have a functional line of occlusion that is tipped down posteriorly and/or an accentuated curve of Spee (Fig. 4.17).

The etiology of a "crooked" smile may be due to "*roll*" of the skeletal maxilla, the maxillary teeth and alveolar process, or an asymmetric elevation of the upper lip. *Roll* of the functional line of occlusion is best visualized on the digital video frame representing the natural unstrained posed social smile (Fig. 4.18).

The intercommissure line is the best frame of reference for evaluation of *roll*. Clinically, the patient with this type of discrepancy will show more tooth mass below the intercommissure line unilaterally as well as more gingival display unilaterally.

Previously, diagnostic imaging techniques were insufficient to visualize discrepancies in maxillomandibular *yaw*. When an orthodontist encountered a major midline shift, a unilateral Class II or Class III molar relationship, or a true unilateral crossbite, they were

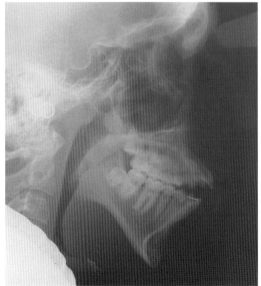

a

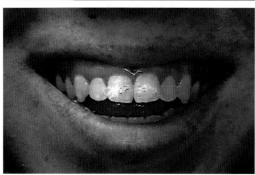

b

Figure 4.17 Patients with an anterior open bite often have a functional line of occlusion that is tipped down posteriorly and/or an accentuated curve of Spee. (**A**) In this particular patient, the lateral radiographic projection clearly shows the accentuated curve of Spee. (**B**) A still frame of the same patient, taken from a digital video clip, illustrates the effect of downward posterior *pitch* on anterior tooth display. Note the increased gingival display in the posterior segments.

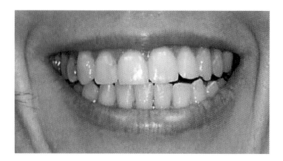

Figure 4.18 *Roll* of the functional line of occlusion is best visualized on the digital video frame representing the natural unstrained posed social smile. The inter-commissure line is the best frame of reference for evaluation of *roll*. Clinically, this patient shows more tooth mass below the intercommissure line on her right side.

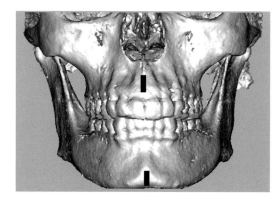

Figure 4.19 The extent of *yaw* can be visualized with three-dimensional imaging and will determine whether treatment involves asymmetric mechanics, asymmetric extractions, unilateral bone anchorage, or orthognathic surgery. In this example, the dental midlines are coincident but an underlying skeletal maxillomandibular yaw exists. (Images courtesy of Imaging Sciences International, Inc., Hatfield, Pennsylvania, and their public relations firm, Gregory FCA Communications, Ardmore, Pennsylvania.)

unable to discern whether maxillomandibular *yaw* was the underlying cause of that discrepancy. Now, the extent of *yaw* can be visualized with three-dimensional imaging and will determine whether treatment involves asymmetric mechanics, asymmetric extractions, unilateral bone anchorage, or orthognathic surgery (Fig. 4.19).

Integration of Imaging into the Clinical Database

The complete clinical database consists of information derived from the doctor–patient interview, direct clinical examination, and diagnostic imaging. In general, the challenge for the orthodontist is to integrate the different data sources and compose a problem-based classification of dentofacial traits. Far too often, orthodontists spend inadequate time on clinical examination and rely heavily on data acquired from diagnostic imaging. To reiterate, the majority of diagnostic data should be taken *directly* from clinical examination. The goal of imaging is to ascertain information about the spatial orientation of dentofacial traits that might not have been possible with use of the human eye alone. At present, imaging technology cannot fully replicate the three-dimensional live patient. The experienced clinician will use the aforementioned imaging techniques to supplement the wealth of data acquired from in vivo examination of the patient.

REFERENCES

Ackerman, J.L., Ackerman, M.B., Brensinger, C.M., Landis, J.R. 1998. A morphometric analysis of the posed smile. *Clin Orthop Res* 1:2–11.

Ackerman, J.L., Proffit, W.R., Sarver, D.M., Ackerman, M.B., Kean, M.R. 2007. Pitch, roll, and yaw: Describing the spatial orientation of dentofacial traits. *Am J Orthod Dentofac Orthop* (in press).

Ackerman, M.B. 2003. Digital video as a clinical tool in orthodontics: Dynamic smile design in diagnosis and treatment planning. In: *29th Annual Moyers Symposium: Information Technology and Orthodontic Treatment, Vol. 40.* Ann Arbor: University of Michigan Press.

Angle, E.H. 1899. Classification of malocclusion. *Dental Cosmos* 41:248–264, 350–357.

Burstone, C.J., Marcotte, M.R. 2000. The treatment occlusal plane. In: *Problem solving in orthodontics: goal-oriented treatment strategies,* pp. 31–50. Chicago: Quintessence Publishing.

Chen, Y., Duan, P., Meng, Y., Chen, X. 2006. Three-dimensional spiral computed tomographic imaging: A new approach to diagnosis and treatment planning of impacted teeth. *Am J Orthod Dentofac Orthop* 130:112–116.

Cohnen, M., Kemper, J., Mobes, O., Pawelzik, J., Modder, U. 2002. Radiation dose in dental radiology. *Eur Radiol* 12:634–637.

Dong, J.K., Jin, T.H., Cho, H.W., Oh, S.C. 1999. The esthetics of the smile: A review of some recent studies. *Int J Prosthodont* 12:9–19.

Ericson, S., Kurol, J. 1988. CT diagnosis of ectopically erupting maxillary canines: A case report. *Eur J Orthod* 10:115–121.

McGlone, C. 2004. *Manual of Photogrammetry,* 5th Edition. Bethesda, Maryland: American Society for Photogrammetry and Remote Sensing.

Moorees, C.F.A., Kean, M.R. 1958. Natural head position, a basic consideration for the analysis of cephalometric radiographs. *Am J Phys Anthrop* 16:213–234.

Morley, J., Eubank, J. 2001. Macroesthetic elements of smile design. *J Am Dent Assoc* 132:39–45.

Scarfe, W.C., Farman, A.G., Sukovic, P. 2006. Clinical applications of cone-beam computed tomography in dental practice. *J Can Dent Assoc* 72:75–80.

Sukovic, P. 2003. Cone beam computed tomography in craniofacial imaging. *Orthod Craniofac Res* 6:31–36.

Classification and Diagnosis of Dentofacial Traits

5

The concept of orthodontic diagnosis has been interpreted in a variety of ways, and consequently the term *diagnosis* has been used by different authors to mean disparate things over the course of modern orthodontic history. Historically, once the orthodontist detected a deviation from Edward Angle's "normal" occlusion, the diagnosis was considered complete (Strang and Thompson 1958). Critics of the traditional Strang approach to orthodontic diagnosis have challenged its very basis (i.e., the Angle classification) and argued that diagnosis must delineate the skeletal versus dental components responsible for variation in dentofacial traits (Case 1921, Hellman 1921, Simon 1926, Broadbent 1937, Brodie 1966, Sassouni 1970). More recently, it has been proposed that diagnosis include not only deviations related to dental and skeletal factors but also the emotional and social ramifications of the patient's orthodontic condition (Moorees and Gron 1966, Ackerman and Proffit 1969). Orthodontic diagnosis during the course of the twentieth century shifted from a somewhat narrow focus (i.e., dental deviations) to what could be termed a more comprehensive assessment of the patient. However, the potential flaw underlying orthodontic diagnosis to date may

be the comparative assessment of a patient's morphology to unscientific normative standards and "imaginary ideals" (Ackerman et al. 2006). Diagnosis in this model implies that any variation from the "ideal" is incompatible with orthodontic health.

Variation in dentofacial traits is usually not indicative of a pathologic process or state of disease per se, and as a result patients rarely complain of somatic symptoms associated with occlusal disharmony. In fact, it is usually the psychological and social ramifications of variation in dentofacial traits that influence a patient's decision to seek orthodontic treatment. To reiterate, if an orthodontic condition is clinically detected by the doctor or perceived by the patient, it must be assessed relative to the patient's three levels of functioning: body part(s), whole person, and the individual in the context of societal values. Diagnosis of a reduction in an individual's state of orthodontic health is determined by the extent of impairment, activity limitation, or participation restriction linked to the specific variation in the dentofacial trait(s). All orthodontic interventions should aim to improve a patient's state of health by diminishing the extent of the disability.

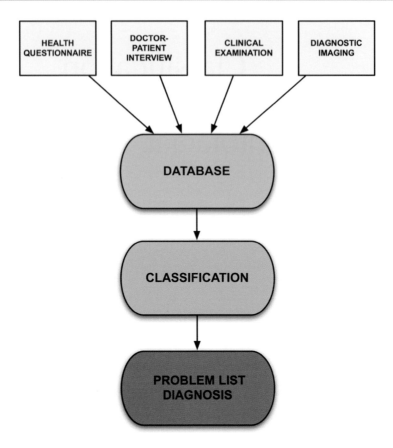

Figure 5.1 The diagnostic process begins with the collection of data concerning the patient's social needs, psychologic status, morphologic attributes, and physiologic functioning. After gathering a comprehensive clinical database, the orthodontist must analyze the data and systematically describe (classify) variation(s) in dentofacial traits that impact the patient's state of orthodontic health. The goal of the diagnostic process in orthodontics is to produce a list of the patient's problems, taking into account the subjective as well as objective findings.

Diagnosis in the enhancement orthodontic model is defined as the task of identifying those variations in dentofacial traits that have brought about a detectable decrement in the patient's health (wellness) as manifested by impairment, activity limitation, or participation restriction. The diagnostic process begins with the collection of data concerning the patient's social needs, psychologic status, morphologic attributes, and physiologic functioning. After gathering a comprehensive clinical database, the orthodontist must analyze the data and systematically describe (classify) variation(s) in dentofacial traits that impact the patient's state of orthodontic health (Fig. 5.1).

The purpose of classification in orthodontic diagnosis is to distill the clinical database into a descriptive list summarizing the patient's problems, that is, those variations in dentofacial traits affecting health, with the required treatment implicit in that description (Table 5.1).

The goal of this chapter is to present a systematic method for the classification of dentofacial traits based on a problem-oriented approach to diagnosis and treatment planning.

Table 5.1

Diagnostic Criterion	Clinical Presentation	Implied Treatment
Angle Class II, division 2 incisor pattern	Flared maxillary lateral incisors, retroclined maxillary central incisors	Level and align maxillary incisors
Short clinical crown height	Insufficient tooth mass vertically, possibly excessive gingival tissue	Clinical crown lengthening and/or extrusion mechanics and/or cosmetic bonding
Maxillary transverse deficiency	Posterior crossbite, narrow palate	Rapid palatal expansion in growing patient, surgery in nongrowing patient
Flat smile arc	Dissonance between curvature of maxillary incisal edges and curvature of lower lip	Differential tooth movement to alter vertical incisor position relative to lower lip

The "Normal" Range of Variation

Natural variation is recognized as a universal basic attribute of the human body; this variation has its beginning in heredity; the compensatory adjustment mechanism fits the variable parts together into a unique morphological unit. Starting with this mosaic individuality, functional adaptation through the dynamic and random forces give the dentofacial complex its specificity by further establishing the individuality of its functional pattern. (Fischer 1952)

In lower species, an arrest of or a delay in development at an embryonic stage is referred to as *neoteny*. The normal period of postnatal dentofacial growth and development in humans is unusually extended compared to nonhuman primates, and this slow pace at which postnatal development occurs is suggestive of neoteny. Specifically, the human neonate remains edentulous for a comparatively long period of time (6 months) with dentitional development spanning roughly 12 years (excluding third molar development). From a phylogenetic point of view, with neoteny came a greater likelihood for morphologic variation, and nowhere is this more apparent than in human dental occlusion (Ackerman and Proffit 1980). The exceedingly long period of dentofacial growth and development in humans permits many external factors to affect the dentofacial complex, and as a result, variation in

dentofacial traits is a normal phenomenon. With that being said, the complex interaction between heredity and environment makes it difficult to assess the relative importance of each in the etiology of variation in dentofacial traits.

Classification in medicine has advanced along both morphologic and etiologic lines, by detection of the organ affected and then, whenever possible, by elucidation of the causative agent. A classification system based on an understanding of etiology has been the ultimate goal of all clinical science (Brash 1956). However, there is one absolute reason why the morphologic approach versus the etiologic approach to classification has prevailed in orthodontics. *Variation in dentofacial traits rarely represents a pathologic state* (Fischer 1952). This is in sharp contrast to the disease entities treated by medicine in which knowledge of the etiology usually provides guidance for treatment. In the absence of an etiologic basis for classifying variation in dentofacial traits, morphologic description is the next best alternative.

Orthodontic Classification

In the late 1960s, Edward Angle's system of orthodontic classification was formally modified from a strictly anteroposterior analysis to include deviations in all three planes of space (Ackerman and Proffit 1969). An orthogonal projection (i.e., a two-dimensional depiction of three-dimensional structures) was used to describe deviation in dentofacial traits. Orthogonal analysis, as this system of classification has come to be known, systematically describes five morphologic characteristics of variation in dentofacial traits and their interrelationships (Fig. 5.2).

When orthogonal analysis was originally proposed nearly 40 years ago, it was conceived according to the prevailing concepts and practices of its day—namely, that ideal occlusion is pivotal for orthodontic health, assessment of appearance is limited to profile analysis, and the three spatial dimensions (sagittal, transverse, and vertical) adequately describe the orientation of dentofacial traits. By today's standards, there are three major flaws in this classification scheme. First, the orthogonal analysis assumed that the most common characteristic (*the universe*) describing all patient's orthodontic conditions was the degree of alignment and symmetry of the teeth and dental arches. Although dental alignment and symmetry is still a common feature in the majority of orthodontic conditions presenting for evaluation, it is *not* the primary criterion affecting orthodontic health. The second major flaw in the orthogonal analysis was that the *only* facet of appearance included in the classification was the assessment of the patient's profile. Today, there is a far greater emphasis on overall facial appearance, anterior tooth display, and their contribution to orthodontic health. Third, the diagnostic imaging techniques of the 1960s did not permit three-dimensional analysis of the orientation of the functional line of occlusion and the esthetic line of the dentition. Contemporary imaging techniques make it possible to describe the exact spatial orientation (e.g., rotation and translation) of these important anatomic features.

Orthogonal Analysis Revisited

The orthogonal analysis has been modified to address the aforementioned shortcomings and to more accurately describe variations in dentofacial traits and their affect on orthodontic health.

The *universe* now represents dentofacial appearance including facial proportions, facial symmetry, facial divergence (profile), smile, and the orientation of the esthetic line of the dentition. Within the universe, the major set describes alignment and symmetry of the teeth and dental arches including whole arch alignment (crowding or spacing), individual tooth position, tooth form, tooth number, periodontal biotype, and the orientation of the functional line of occlusion. Three interlocking subsets within this major set describe transverse, sagittal, and vertical deviations. Any orthodontic condition can be sufficiently described by five or fewer characteristics (Fig. 5.3).

Classification Procedure

Step 1: Appearance Evaluation (Fig. 5.4)

The first step in classification is to evaluate the patient's dentofacial appearance. The majority of data regarding appearance were collected during the doctor–patient interview and the global and regional levels of clinical appraisal. Digital videography will provide supplemental information related to the dynamics of anterior tooth display. Variations in facial proportion, facial symmetry, facial divergence (profile), smile, and the orientation of the esthetic line of the dentition are described in the category of appearance. A descriptive list summarizing the patient's problems related to appearance should be generated.

Appearance Terminology
- *Facial proportion*: For example, long lower face, short lower face, midface deficiency (anteroposterior), vertical maxillary excess,

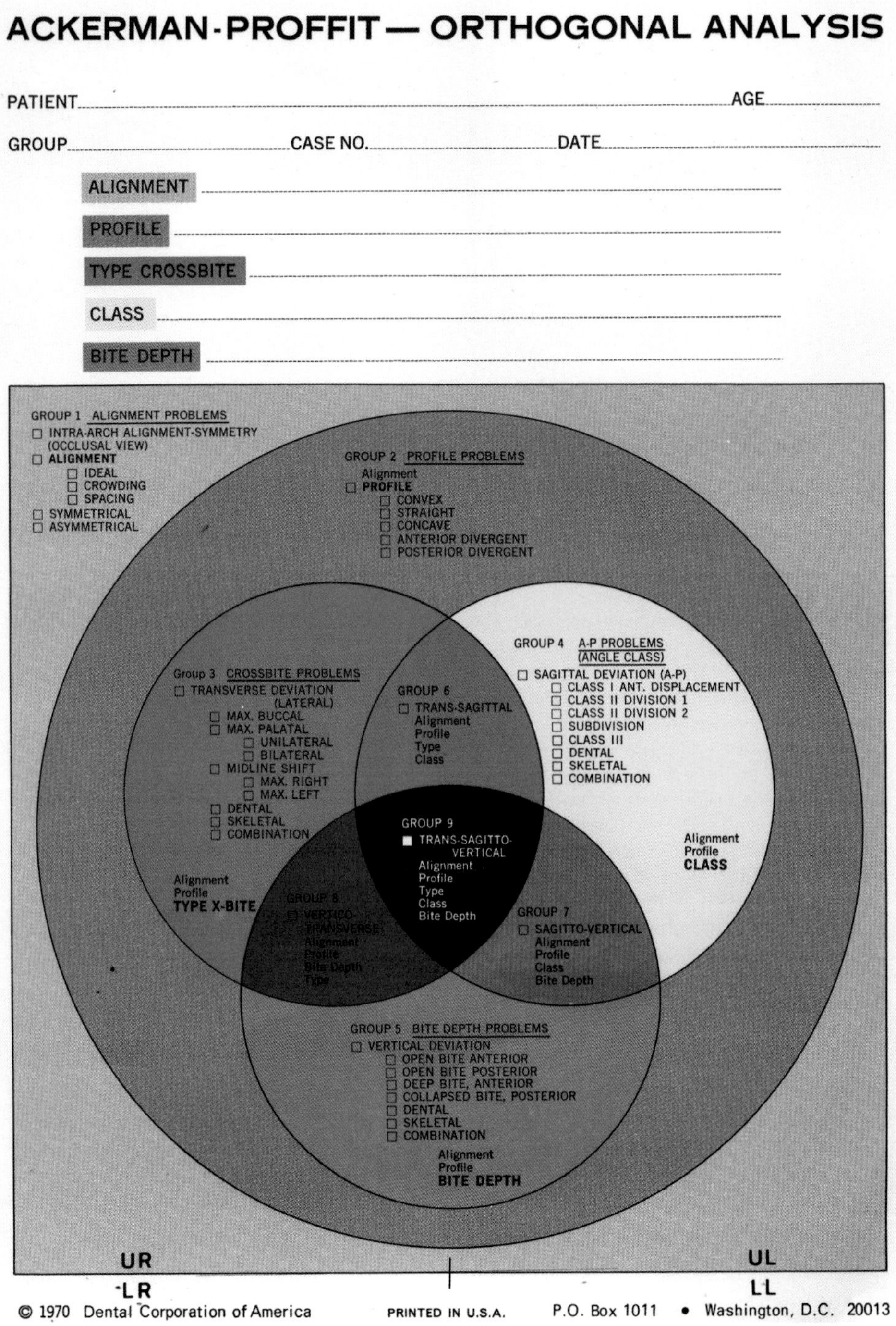

Figure 5.2 The original Ackerman-Proffit orthogonal analysis. (Image courtesy of Dr. James L. Ackerman; the concept was originally presented in Ackerman, J.L., Proffit, W.R. 1969. The characteristics of malocclusion: A modern approach to classification and diagnosis. *Am J Orthod* 56:443–454.)

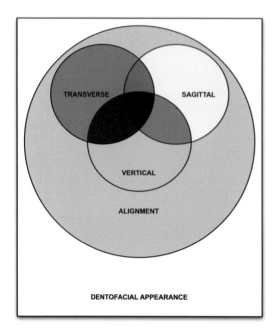

Figure 5.3 The modified orthogonal analysis. The orthogonal analysis has been modified to more accurately describe variations in dentofacial traits and their affect on orthodontic health. The *universe* now represents dentofacial appearance including facial proportions, facial symmetry, facial divergence (profile), smile, and the orientation of the esthetic line of the dentition. Within the universe, the major set describes alignment and symmetry of the teeth and dental arches including whole arch alignment (crowding or spacing), individual tooth position, tooth form, tooth number, periodontal biotype, and the orientation of the functional line of occlusion. Three interlocking subsets within this major set describe transverse, sagittal, and vertical deviations. Any orthodontic condition can be sufficiently described by five or fewer characteristics.

excessive chin height, vertical maxillary deficiency, diminished chin height, narrow midface, narrow lower facial third, wide alar base, narrow alar base, lip incompetence, deepened nasolabial folds.

- *Facial symmetry/asymmetry*: For example, nasal asymmetry, mandibular asymmetry, chin asymmetry, asymmetric dental midlines.
- *Facial convexity/concavity*: For example, excessive nasal projection, acute nasolabial angle, obtuse nasolabial angle, excessive lip eversion, obliterated labiomental sulcus.

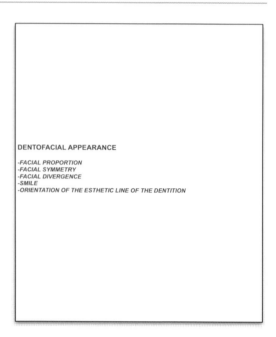

Figure 5.4 Appearance evaluation.

- *Facial divergence*: For example, orthognathic, posteriorly divergent, anteriorly divergent, insufficient chin projection, excessive chin projection.
- *Anterior tooth display/smile*: For example, excessive tooth display at rest or smile, insufficient tooth display at rest or smile, excessive gingival display at rest or smile, insufficient gingival display at rest or smile, reverse resting lip line, flat smile arc, reverse smile arc, excessive buccal corridor, excessively flared incisors, severely retroclined incisors.
- *Orientation of the esthetic line of the dentition*: For example, pitch up or down, anteriorly or posteriorly, roll up or down on one side or the other, and yaw to one side or the other about the vertical axis.

Step 2: Alignment Evaluation (Fig. 5.5)

The second step in classification is the assessment of alignment and symmetry of the teeth and dental arches. This is accomplished through clinical appraisal at the local level, modeling of the dentition, and radiographic imaging of the dentition. Variations in whole

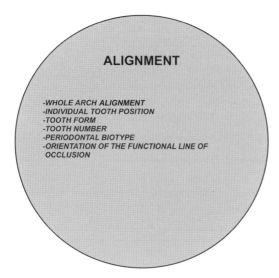

Figure 5.5 Alignment evaluation.

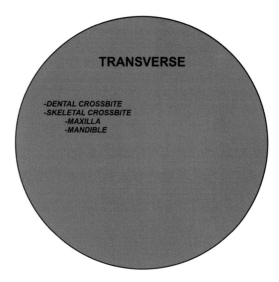

Figure 5.6 Transverse evaluation.

arch alignment, individual tooth position, tooth form, tooth number, periodontal biotype, and the orientation of the functional line of occlusion are described in the category of alignment. A descriptive list summarizing the patient's problems related to alignment should be generated.

Alignment Terminology
- *Whole arch alignment*: For example, crowding or spacing.
- *Individual tooth position*: For example, labioversion, lingualversion, buccoversion, palatoversion, palatal impaction, labial impaction, transposition, transmigration, ectopic eruption.
- *Tooth form*: For example, short clinical crown height, peg-shaped lateral incisors, mottled enamel, excessive tooth wear.
- *Tooth number*: For example, congenitally missing tooth or teeth, supernumerary tooth or teeth, fusion, gemination.
- *Periodontal biotype*: For example, thick/flat, thin/scalloped, and pronounced thin/scalloped.
- *Orientation of the functional line of occlusion*: For example, pitch up or down, anteriorly or posteriorly, roll up or down on one side or the other, and yaw to one side or the other about the vertical axis.

Step 3: Transverse Evaluation (Fig. 5.6)

The third step in classification is the assessment of the patient's dental arches and skeletal bases with regard to variation in the transverse dimension. Specifically, the buccolingual relationships of the posterior teeth are described. This is accomplished through clinical appraisal at the global, regional, and local levels and the analysis of the models of the dentition (plaster or digital). A judgment has to be made as to whether the deviation is dentoalveolar in nature or skeletal in nature or due to a combination of the two. Most transverse problems have components of both, with one or the other predominating. For example, if a bilateral palatal crossbite exists, the clinician must ask whether the problem is a narrow maxilla or a narrow dental arch although the skeletal width is correct. As a general rule, "maxillary" and "mandibular" are used to indicate where the problem is located. Maxillary palatal crossbite implies a narrow maxillary arch, while mandibular buccal crossbite indicates excess mandibular width. A descriptive list summarizing the patient's problems related to transverse deviations should be generated.

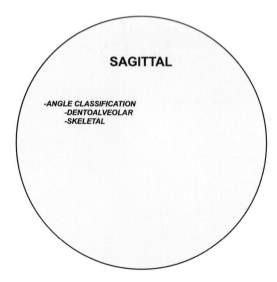

Figure 5.7 Sagittal evaluation.

Transverse Terminology

- *Crossbite (skeletal, dental, or combination)*: For example, unilateral maxillary palatal crossbite, bilateral maxillary palatal crossbite, unilateral maxillary buccal crossbite, bilateral maxillary buccal crossbite, unilateral mandibular buccal crossbite, bilateral mandibular buccal crossbite, unilateral mandibular lingual crossbite, bilateral mandibular lingual crossbite.
- *Inclination of teeth in buccal segments*: For example, flared labially, inclined palatally (upper), or inclined lingually (lower).
- *Roll*: For example, maxillary (dental or skeletal) or mandibular (dental or skeletal).

Step 4: Sagittal (Anteroposterior) Evaluation (Fig. 5.7)

The fourth step in classification is the assessment of the patient's dental arches and skeletal bases with regard to variation in the sagittal (anteroposterior) dimension. This is accomplished through clinical appraisal at the global, regional and local levels and the analysis of diagnostic imaging. The Angle Classification is used and supplemented with the descriptor "skeletal," "dentoalveolar," or

a combination. In the case of Angle Class II and Class III deviations, the clinician should note whether the maxilla, the mandible, or a combination of both contributes to the specific morphologic problem. A descriptive list summarizing the patient's problems related to sagittal deviations should be generated.

Sagittal Terminology

- *Angle Class (skeletal, dental, or combination and maxilla or mandible)*: For example, Class I, Class I with excessive overjet, Class I with anterior crossbite, Class II–Division 1 (maxillary protrusion), Class II–Division 1 (mandibular retrognathia), Class II–Division 1 (combination), Class II–Division 2 (maxillary protrusion), Class II–Division 2 (mandibular retrognathia), Class II–Division 2 (combination), Class II–Division 1 Subdivision (maxillary yaw), Class II–Division 1 Subdivision (mandibular yaw), Class II–Division 2 Subdivision (maxillary yaw), Class II–Division 2 Subdivision (mandibular yaw), Class III with anterior crossbite, Class III (maxillary retrusion), Class III (mandibular prognathism), Class III Subdivision (maxillary yaw), Class III Subdivision (mandibular yaw).

Step 5: Vertical Evaluation (Fig. 5.8)

The fifth step in classification is the assessment of the patient's dental arches and skeletal bases with regard to variation in the vertical dimension. This is accomplished through clinical appraisal at the global, regional, and local levels and the analysis of diagnostic imaging. *Bite depth* is used to describe the vertical relationships. The possibilities are anterior open bite, anterior deep bite, posterior open bite, or posterior collapsed bite. The clinician must determine whether deviations are skeletal, dentoalveolar, or a combination of both. A descriptive list summarizing the patient's problems related to vertical deviations should be generated.

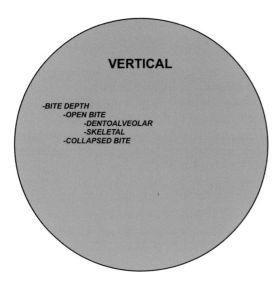

Figure 5.8 Vertical evaluation.

Vertical Terminology

- *Bite depth (skeletal, dental, or combination)*: For example, anterior open bite, anterior deep bite, posterior open bite, or posterior collapsed bite.
- *Pitch*: For example, anterior maxilla up, anterior maxilla down, posterior maxilla down, posterior maxilla down.

Problem-Oriented Diagnosis and Treatment Planning

The goal of the diagnostic process in enhancement orthodontics is to produce a list of the patient's problems, taking into account subjective as well as objective findings. This cognitive exercise is a modification of the problem-oriented approach to medical records (Weed 1969, 2004). In this approach, the treatment plan is the connecting link between diagnosis and therapy in which the orthodontist constructs a working strategy for resolving the patient's problems. Orthodontic treatment is to diagnosis what the experiment is to a research hypothesis (Ackerman and Proffit 1975). The clinical

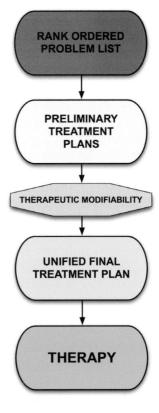

Figure 5.9 In the treatment planning regimen, the orthodontist must (1) generate a comprehensive problem list, rank ordered according to the patient's preferences; (2) propose treatment plans for each of the ranked problems; and then (3) synthesize the preliminary treatment plans into a unified final treatment plan. Each problem should be evaluated relative to its therapeutic modifiability.

result either supports or rejects the orthodontist's diagnosis.

The veteran orthodontist, when faced with common variations in dentofacial traits, begins to interpret his or her findings during the clinical examination, labels them through classification, and constructs preliminary treatment plans almost instinctively. In the treatment planning regimen, the clinician must (1) generate a comprehensive problem list that is rank ordered according to the patient's preferences, (2) propose preliminary treatment plans for each of the ranked problems, and then (3) synthesize the preliminary treatment plans into a unified final treatment plan (Fig. 5.9).

The first stage of decision-making is a process called *knowledge coupling*, which is matching specific patient data with general orthodontic knowledge (Weed 1999). For each patient problem, three requirements must be satisfied in that coupling process. First, in retrieving general orthodontic knowledge, all variables relevant to diagnostic problems and all treatment alternatives must be taken into account. Atypical characteristics and nonstandard treatments potentially relevant to unique patients must not be excluded from consideration based simply on case reports in the orthodontic literature or a clinician's experience with other patients. Second, in retrieving patient-specific data, the maximum amount of available information that discriminates among the relevant variation in dentofacial traits should be collected prior to treatment, in order to classify patient uniqueness. Third, the linkages between the first two requirements must be identified in the coupling process, so that the therapeutic implications of variation in the patient's dentofacial appearance will be readily perceivable to the clinician and patient when they meet to select the most desirable treatment plan in the second stage of decision-making.

Therapeutic Modifiability

Each preliminary treatment plan should be assessed relative to therapeutic modifiability. *Therapeutic modifiability* (Moorees and Gron 1966) refers to the clinician's ability to predict the "achievable optimum" for a patient when attempting to satisfy the treatment objectives of a given preliminary treatment plan. The greater the effort needed to produce a small improvement in a dentofacial trait, the lesser the therapeutic modifiability, and vice versa. Once the problem list has been ordered relative to therapeutic modifiability, reasonable treatment goals can be set and a unified final treatment plan synthesized.

Treatment Planning and the Dimension of Time

When evaluating therapeutic modifiability, the clinician must also consider two points in time: (1) the completion of active treatment and (2) the cessation of orthodontic retention. The first question the clinician must ask when planning tooth movement and/or jaw surgery is how stable will the correction be at the completion of active treatment. The second question that should be asked is what will most likely occur when the patient stops complying with the prescribed plan of retention. Currently, it is nearly impossible to predict the *timing, degree,* and *direction* of relapse for many dentofacial traits. Traditionally, orthodontists have argued that when the teeth are knowingly moved into "unstable" positions, they will ultimately experience rebound or physiologic recovery (Horowitz and Hixon 1969). However, *all* orthodontic movements are to some extent "unstable."

Many tooth-related postretention changes are due to normal maturational changes in the dentofacial complex. The resting pressures of the tongue, lips, and forces created within the periodontal ligament contribute to the multifactorial etiology of relapse (Proffit 1978). Because the nature of orthodontic relapse is not entirely known or predictable (Melrose and Millett 1998, Littlewood et al. 2006), patients should be advised that lifetime retention is needed to maintain tooth position. Nowhere is this more evident than in the case of lower incisor crowding (Ormiston et al. 2005). The orthodontist, in order to satisfy the tenets of informed consent, should discuss, when possible, the short- and long-term prognoses for proposed modification of a dentofacial trait or traits.

Therapeutic Diagnosis

No orthodontic treatment plan should be considered written in stone. That is to say, mid-course corrections are often made during orthodontic therapy based on treatment response, patient cooperation, growth, or any unforeseen events. Therapeutic diagnosis is defined as a procedure in which an initial diagnosis is made in the face of some uncertainty as to the nature of the problem (Ackerman and Proffit 1970). The first stage of treatment is based specifically on this tentative diagnosis, and the response to treatment is used to confirm or reject the original diagnosis. For example, a moderate to severe arch perimeter deficiency in both arches may be diagnosed as a result of arch constriction. Consequently, a nonextraction treatment approach is selected. If after the leveling and aligning phase of treatment the teeth are positioned appropriately along the functional line of occlusion with an improvement in dentofacial appearance, the original diagnosis is supported. However, if crowding persists or the tooth movement has negatively affected dentofacial appearance (e.g., expansion beyond the limits of the soft tissue envelope), the diagnosis will have to be modified, perhaps to include a tooth size/arch size discrepancy, and the extraction of premolar teeth should be considered.

Therapeutic diagnosis is not a substitute for systematic classification and the aforementioned diagnosis and treatment-planning regimen. It also should not be used to conceal poor logic or fuzzy thinking. A definitive orthodontic treatment plan can be implemented *only* after a definitive diagnosis has been made. In some orthodontic conditions, it is *not* possible to make a definitive diagnosis prior to commencing therapy. Treatment response in these cases will confirm or reject the original diagnosis and establish the final treatment plan.

See Figures 5.10, 5.11, and 5.12.

Age

Twenty years, 9 months

Chief Concern

"My upper teeth are going back."

Medical History

Four eye surgeries between 15 months and 6 years of age.

Dental History

Oral hygiene within normal limits
Low caries rate
Dental visits at 6-month intervals

Orthogonal Analysis

Dentofacial Appearance

Downward anterior pitch of the esthetic line of the dentition
Excessive gingival display
Excessive buccal corridor
Nonconsonant smile arc
Excessive nasal projection

Alignment

Excessive retroclination of maxillary and mandibular incisors
Mandibular arch perimeter deficiency
Downward anterior pitch of the functional line of occlusion with a reverse curve of Spee in the maxillary arch
Square arch forms

Transverse

Excessive palatal inclination of maxillary canines, premolars, and molars
Excessive lingual inclination of mandibular canines, premolars, and molars

Sagittal

No deviation

Vertical

Anterior deep bite.

Problem List (Rank Ordered by Patient Preferences)

1. Excessive retroclination of incisors
2. Excessive inclination of buccal segments
3. Excessive buccal corridor
4. Excessive gingival display
5. Downward anterior pitch of the esthetic line of the dentition and functional line of occlusion
6. Nonconsonant smile arc
7. Square arch forms
8. Mandibular arch perimeter deficiency
9. Anterior deep bite
10. Excessive nasal projection (not perceived by patient)

Preliminary Treatment Plans

Problem 1: Correct labiolingual torque of incisors
Problem 2: Correct labiolingual torque of buccal segments
Problem 3: Lateral movement of tooth mass into buccal corridor via torque and change in arch form

Problem 4: Intrusion during leveling and aligning, Gingivectomy and clinical crown lengthening

Problem 5: Leveling of curve of Spee

Problem 6: Differential bracket placement for appropriate incisal edge position

Problem 7: Application of a catenary arch form (*catenary* refers to the shape that a loop of chain would take if it were suspended from two hooks the length of the chain and the width between the supports will determine the exact shape of the curve)

Problem 8: Gain space through arch expansion and change in arch form

Problem 9: Bite opening mechanics, leveling curve of Spee

Problem 10: Rhinoplasty

Unified Final Treatment Plan

Level and align maxillary and mandibular arches

Create coordinated catenary arch forms

Improve anterior tooth display (incisor display, buccal corridor, gingival display, and smile arc)

Improve overbite–overjet relationship

Therapy

Modified straight wire appliance

Direct bond ↑↓ fixed appliances (including second molars)

Successive leveling archwires

Working movements (application of torque)

Interarch elastics if needed

Gingivectomy and/or clinical crown lengthening if appropriate

Retention

Maxillary Hawley retainer

Fixed lingual canine-to-canine retainer bonded to each tooth (No. 22 to No. 27)

Mandibular Hawley retainer to be worn over the fixed retainer (to maintain posterior arch width)

Commentary

This patient illustrates variation in the principal dentofacial traits composing the appearance of the smile (e.g., incisor display, gingival display, buccal corridor, arch form, and smile arc). Although clinical examination revealed excessive nasal projection in profile view, a discussion with the patient confirmed that this variation had little effect on her self-concept and wellness. That is why it is ranked low on the problem list and was not incorporated in the final unified treatment plan.

The tentative diagnosis of excessive gingival display due to the downward anterior pitch of the esthetic line of the dentition and functional line of occlusion will be tested during the initial phase of treatment. If bite-opening mechanics diminish the amount of gingival display at smile, then the original diagnosis is confirmed. However, if there is still gingival display after the teeth are leveled and aligned, then other factors such as excessive upper lip animation or short clinical crowns should be considered. At that point, gingivectomy and clinical crown lengthening would be an option.

Chief Concern _{upper} teeth are going back

Reason for seeking orthodontic advice:
[✓] Information
[ ] Treatment at this time
[ ] Clarification of previously received information or conflicting information
[ ] Continuation of treatment

Figure 5.10 The patient's chief concern and reason for seeking orthodontic advice.

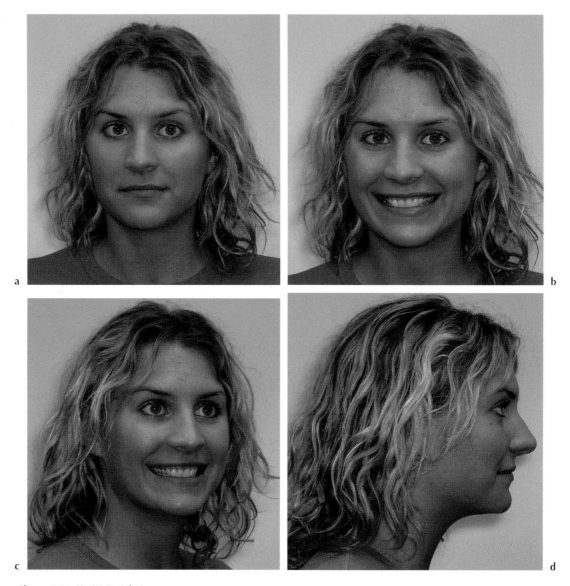

a
b
c
d

Figure 5.11 (A–D) Facial views.

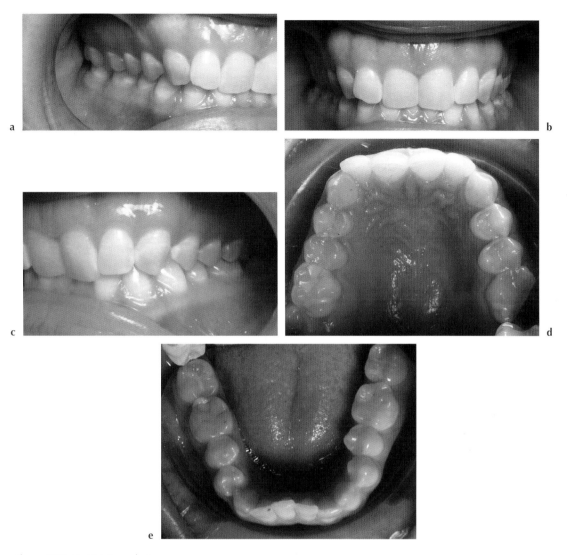

Figure 5.12 (**A–E**) Intraoral views.

See Figures 5.13, 5.14, and 5.15.

Age

Eleven years

Chief Concern

The parent and patient did not indicate a chief concern on the health questionnaire. In the course of the doctor–patient interview, it became clear that the parents were seeking orthodontic advice on the recommendation of the dentist. His concern was the supernumerary mandibular incisor.

Medical History

Noncontributory

Dental History

Oral hygiene within normal limits
Low caries rate
Dental visits at 6-month intervals

Orthogonal Analysis

Dentofacial Appearance

No deviation

Alignment

Supernumerary mandibular incisor
Small-sized maxillary lateral incisors
Maxillary spacing
Mild rotation of mandibular incisors

Transverse

No deviation

Sagittal

No deviation

Vertical

No deviation

Problem List (No Patient Preferences)

1. Supernumerary mandibular incisor
2. Small-sized maxillary lateral incisors
3. Maxillary spacing
4. Mild rotation of mandibular incisors

Preliminary Treatment Plans

Problem 1: Extract supernumerary incisor
Problem 2: Cosmetic dentistry to improve tooth form
Problem 3: Orthodontically condense posterior space
Problem 4: Level and align mandibular teeth, gain space with reproximation

Unified Final Treatment Plan

No orthodontic treatment indicated
Recommend mandibular Hawley retainer, nighttime only
Cosmetic dentistry for the small-sized maxillary lateral incisors at a later stage of maturation

Commentary

This patient illustrates variation in tooth number and tooth size. From a maturational standpoint, he was just beginning the puberal growth spurt and his dental age was several months ahead of his chronologic age. A consistent facial growth trend was anticipated. The last permanent maxillary premolar was within weeks of eruption, and all the permanent teeth drifted vertically into occlusion within 3 months.

At this point in time, the patient and his parents had no chief concern related to dentofacial appearance or function. In fact, they were quite happy with the look of his smile. The discussion in the doctor–patient/parent conference focused on management of the supernumerary mandibular incisor. The following options were presented:

1. Extract the supernumerary incisor
   Level and align the mandibular arch, condense residual space

Cosmetic dentistry for the small-sized maxillary lateral incisors at a later stage of maturation
2. Leave the supernumerary incisor in place
   Reproximate to gain arch perimeter
   Level and align the mandibular arch
   Cosmetic dentistry for the small-sized maxillary lateral incisors at a later stage of maturation
3. No orthodontic treatment
   Fabricate a mandibular Hawley retainer to prevent further rotations
   Cosmetic dentistry for the small-sized maxillary lateral incisors at a later stage of maturation

From a therapeutic modifiability standpoint, the parents correctly concluded that the first two options required a great amount of effort for very little change in dentofacial appearance and orthodontic health. Therefore, the third option was selected.

PSYCHOSOCIAL AND PHYSICAL GROWTH STATUS

Chief Concern _____

Reason for seeking orthodontic advice:
[✓] Information
[ ] Treatment at this time
[ ] Clarification of previously received information or conflicting information
[ ] Continuation of treatment

Figure 5.13 The patient's chief concern and reason for seeking orthodontic advice.

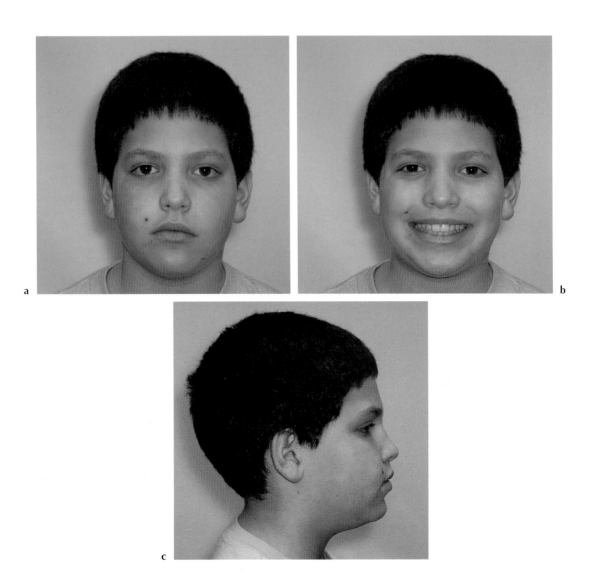

Figure 5.14 (**A–C**) Facial views.

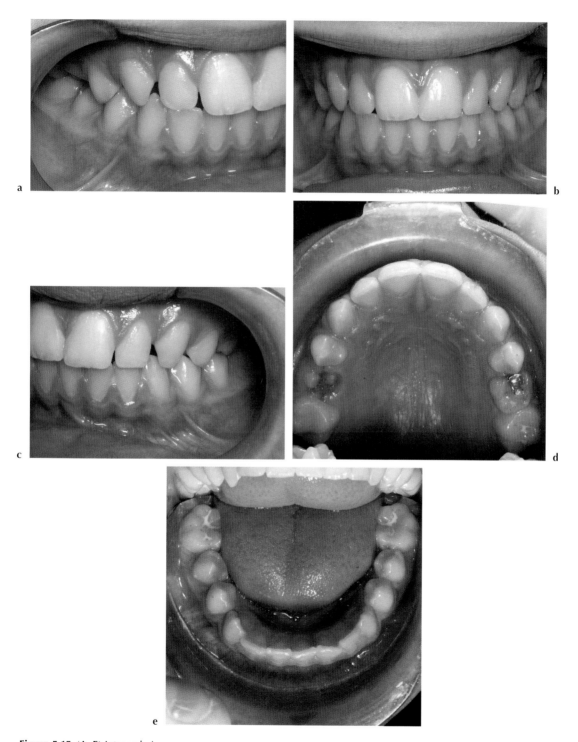

Figure 5.15 (A–E) Intraoral views.

REFERENCES

Ackerman, J.L., Proffit, W.R. 1969. The characteristics of malocclusion: A modern approach to classification and diagnosis. *Am J Orthod* 56:443–454.

Ackerman, J.L., Proffit, W.R. 1970. Treatment response as an aid in diagnosis and treatment planning. *Am J Orthod* 57:490–496.

Ackerman, J.L., Proffit, W.R. 1975. Diagnosis and planning treatment in orthodontics. In: *Current orthodontic concepts and techniques,* 2nd Edition, edited by T.M. Graber and B.F. Swain. Philadelphia: W.B. Saunders Company.

Ackerman, J.L., Proffit, W.R. 1980. Preventive and interceptive orthodontics: A strong theory proves weak in practice. *Angle Orthod* 50:75–87.

Ackerman, M.B., Rinchuse, D.J., Rinchuse, D.J. 2006. ABO certification in the age of evidence and enhancement. *Am J Orthod Dentofac Orthop* 130:133–140.

Brash, J.C. 1956. *The aetiology of irregularity and malocclusion of the teeth.* London: Dental Board of the United Kingdom.

Broadbent, B.H. 1937. The face of the normal child. *Angle Orthod* 7:183–208.

Brodie, A.G. 1966. The apical base: Zone of interaction between the intestinal and skeletal system. *Angle Orthod* 36:136–151.

Case, C.S. 1921. *A practical treatise on the techniques and principles of dental orthopedia and prosthetic correction of cleft palate.* Chicago: C.S. Case Company.

Feinstein, A.R. 1963. Boolean algebra and clinical taxonomy. *N Engl J Med* 269:929–938.

Fischer, B. 1952. *Orthodontics: Diagnosis, prognosis, treatment,* p. 44, Philadelphia: W.B. Saunders Company.

Hellman, M. 1921. Variations in occlusion. *Dental Cosmos* 63:608–619.

Horowitz, S.L., Hixon, E.H. 1969. Physiologic recovery following orthodontic treatment. *Am J Orthod* 55:1–4.

Littlewood, S.J., Millett, D.T., Doubleday, B., Bearn, D.R., Worthington, H.V. 2006. Retention procedures for stablising tooth position after treatment with orthodontic braces. *Cochrane Database Syst Rev* 25:CD002283.

Melrose, C., Millett, D.T. 1998. Toward a perspective on orthodontic retention? *Am J Orthod Dentofac Orthop* 113:507–514.

Moorees, C.F.A., Gron, A.M. 1966. Principles of orthodontic diagnosis. *Angle Orthod* 36:258–262.

Ormiston, J.P., Huang, G.J., Little, R.M., Decker, J.D., Seuk, G.D. 2005. Retrospective analysis of long-term stable and unstable orthodontic treatment outcomes. *Am J Orthod Dentofac Orthop* 128:568–574.

Proffit, W.R. 1978. Equilibrium theory revisited: Factors influencing position of the teeth. *Angle Orthod* 48:175–186.

Sassouni, V. 1970. The Class II syndrome: Differential diagnosis and treatment. *Angle Orthod* 40:334–341.

Simon, P. 1926. *Fundamental principles of a systematic diagnosis of dental anomalies.* Translated by B.E. Lischer. Boston: Stratford Company.

Strang, R.H., Thompson, W.M. 1958. *A textbook of orthodontia,* 4th Edition. Philadelphia: Lea & Febiger.

Weed, L.L. 1969. *Medical records, medical education and patient care: The problem-oriented record as a basic tool.* Cleveland, Ohio: Case Western Reserve Press.

Weed, L.L. 1999. Clinical judgment revisited. *Method Inform Med* 38:279–286.

Weed, L.L. 2004. Shedding our illusions: A better way of medicine. *Sexual Reprod Menopause* 2:45–52.

Beyond Normal: Enhancement of Dentofacial Traits

6

The scope of enhancement orthodontics ranges from the treatment of a single dentofacial trait to the "extreme makeover" of dentofacial appearance involving plastic and reconstructive surgery, orthognathic surgery, orthodontics, periodontics, and advanced cosmetic dentistry. The following 10 case studies illustrate a spectrum of enhancements seen in everyday orthodontic practice. All of the patients had some recognizable variation in a dentofacial trait or traits, which affected their functioning in a social context and caused a decrement in their state of orthodontic health (wellness). Enhancement orthodontic outcome is detailed in a three-step process. First, the primary characteristic (orthogonal analysis) of the orthodontic problem is listed. Second, the specific variation in the dentofacial trait is described. Third, the method and type of enhancement used are enumerated.

Case Study 6.1

See Figures 6.1 through 6.6 and Table 6.1.

Orthogonal Analysis

See Table 6.2.

Problem List (Rank Ordered by Patient Preferences)

Labioverted maxillary left permanent lateral incisor (tooth No. 10)
Mild mandibular arch perimeter deficiency

Treatment Options

1. Level and align maxillary and mandibular arches
2. Level and align maxillary arch
   Mandibular Hawley retainer to prevent continued crowding
3. No treatment

Unified Final Treatment Plan

Level and align maxillary arch
Mandibular Hawley retainer to be worn at night only

Therapy

Modified straight wire appliance
Direct bond ↑ fixed appliance (first molar to first molar)
Successive leveling archwires

Actual Treatment Time

Four months

Retention

Direct bond palatal wire between tooth No. 9 and tooth No. 10
Maxillary Hawley retainer to be worn at night only
Mandibular Hawley retainer to be worn at night only

Enhancement Outcome

See Table 6.3.

Commentary

This patient's chief concern was limited to a variation in one well-defined dentofacial trait. The labioverted maxillary left permanent lateral incisor (tooth No. 10) was negatively affecting incisor display. Limited orthodontic treatment was utilized to align tooth No. 10, improving the appearance of the patient's smile. It was explained to the patient that the fixed palatal wire between tooth No. 9 and tooth No. 10 should remain in place for an indefinite period of time.

PSYCHOSOCIAL AND PHYSICAL GROWTH STATUS

Chief Concern: _Cosmetic – (alignment + ~~teeth~~ color)_

Reason for seeking orthodontic advice:

[✓] Information
[ ] Treatment at this time
[ ] Clarification of previously received information or conflicting information
[ ] Continuation of treatment

Figure 6.1 The patient's chief concern and reason for seeking orthodontic advice.

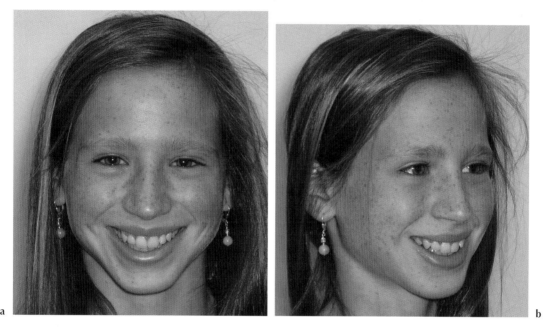

a   b

Figure 6.2 (**A**) Facial view during social smile. (**B**) Three-quarter facial view during social smile. Note the labioverted maxillary left permanent lateral incisor (tooth No. 10).

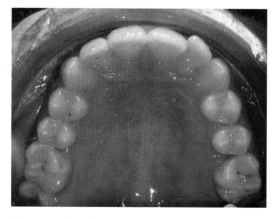

Figure 6.3 Maxillary occlusal view.

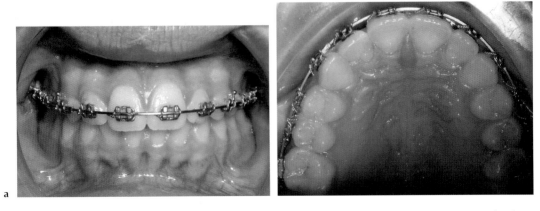

Figure 6.4 Tooth No. 10 has been leveled and aligned via maxillary fixed appliance therapy. (**A**) Front occlusal view. (**B**) Maxillary occlusal view.

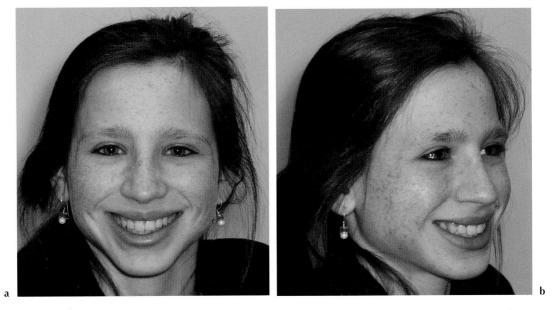

Figure 6.5 Post-treatment. (**A**) Facial view during social smile. (**B**) Three-quarter facial view during social smile.

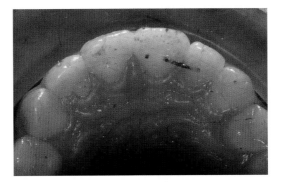

Figure 6.6 A bonded palatal wire between tooth No. 9 and tooth No. 10 is an adjunct to the removable Hawley retainer prescribed for the patient. Tooth No. 10 will require indefinite retention.

Table 6.1 Patient Data

Age	13 Years, 7 months
Chief complaint	"Cosmetic—alignment and color"
Medical history	Hypothyroid, takes Synthroid Pyelonephritis
Dental history	Oral hygiene within normal limits
	Low caries rate
	Dental visits at 6-month intervals

Table 6.2 Orthognal Analysis

Dentofacial appearance	Maxillary left permanent lateral incisor (tooth No. 10) negatively affecting anterior tooth display
Alignment	Labioverted maxillary left permanent lateral incisor (tooth No. 10)
	Mild mandibular arch perimeter deficiency
Transverse	No deviation
Sagittal	No deviation
Vertical	No deviation

Table 6.3 Enhancement Outcome

Primary Characteristic	Specific Variation	Enhancement
Dentofacial appearance	Unattractive anterior tooth display (labioverted tooth No. 10)	Anterior tooth display improved through alignment of tooth No. 10
Alignment	Labioverted tooth No. 10	Aligned tooth No. 10

Case Study 6.2

See Figures 6.7 through 6.12 and Table 6.4.

Orthogonal Analysis

See Table 6.5.

Problem List (Rank Ordered by Patient Preferences)

Mild mandibular arch perimeter deficiency
Maxillary diastemata
Butterfly maxillary permanent central incisors

Treatment Options

1. Level and align maxillary arch
   Condense space in maxillary arch
   Level and align mandibular arch
2. Level and align mandibular arch
3. No treatment

Unified Final Treatment Plan

Level and align maxillary arch
Condense space in maxillary arch
Level and align mandibular arch

Therapy

Modified straight wire appliance
Direct bond ↑↓ limited fixed appliances (2 × 6, canine-to-canine and first molars)
Successive leveling archwires
Working movement (elastomeric thread to close space)

Actual Treatment Time

Six months

Retention

Direct bond palatal wire between tooth No. 8 and tooth No. 9
Maxillary Hawley retainer to be worn at night only
Fixed lingual canine-to-canine retainer bonded to each tooth (No. 22 to No. 27)

Enhancement Outcome

See Table 6.6.

Commentary

This patient was referred to the orthodontist for assessment of crowding in the anterior portion of the mandibular arch. Her dentist had noted an increase in crowding during the second transitional period of dentitional development. In the doctor–patient interview, the patient expressed more concern over the progressive crowding than the maxillary diastemata. After weighing all of the information provided to her at the doctor–patient conference, the patient and parent decided to address both the mandibular crowding and the maxillary spacing.

When closing diastemata, an assessment of the patient's periodontal biotype is critical. In this case, the patient had a thick/flat periodontal biotype. Tooth contacts in this biotype are broader both incisogingivally

Beyond Normal: Enhancement of Dentofacial Traits 91

and faciolingually. This anatomic feature facilitated space closure without the appearance of a "black triangle" incisal to the interdental papilla between tooth No. 8 and tooth No. 9. The frenum attachment in this case did not require resection. It was explained to the patient that space closure in orthodontics is a very unstable type of tooth movement. As a result, it was recommended that the fixed palatal wire between tooth No. 8 and tooth No. 9 remain in place for an indefinite period of time.

PSYCHOSOCIAL AND PHYSICAL GROWTH STATUS

Chief Concern: _TEETH CROWDING_

Reason for seeking orthodontic advice:

[✓] Information
[✓] Treatment at this time
[ ] Clarification of previously received information or conflicting information
[ ] Continuation of treatment

Figure 6.7 The patient's chief concern and reason for seeking orthodontic advice.

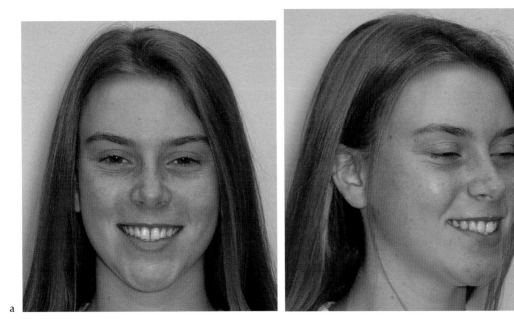

a   b

Figure 6.8 (**A**) Facial view during social smile. (**B**) Three-quarter facial view during social smile. Note the butterfly pattern of the maxillary right and left permanent central incisors (teeth No. 8 and No. 9).

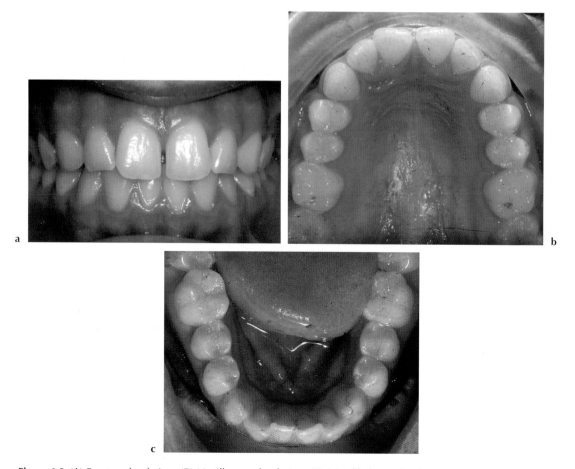

Figure 6.9 (**A**) Front occlusal view. (**B**) Maxillary occlusal view. (**C**) Mandibular occlusal view.

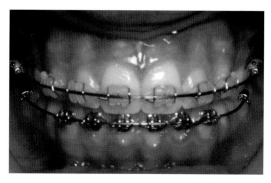

Figure 6.10 Maxillary and mandibular limited fixed appliances in place. The maxillary midline diastema has been closed. Note the development of an interdental gingival papilla between teeth No. 8 and No. 9.

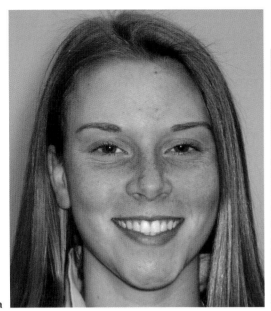
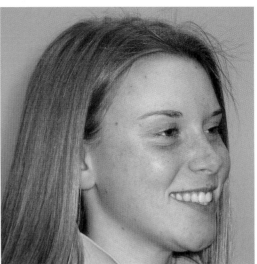

a
b

Figure 6.11 Post-treatment. (**A**) Facial view during social smile. (**B**) Three-quarter facial view during social smile.

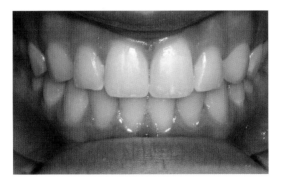

Figure 6.12 Post-treatment front occlusal view.

Table 6.4 Patient Data

Age	13 Years, 8 months
Chief complaint	"Teeth crowding"
Medical history	Noncontributory
Dental history	Oral hygiene within normal limits
	Low caries rate
	Dental visits at 6-month intervals

Table 6.5 Orthognal Analysis

Dentofacial appearance	Prominent maxillary midline diastema negatively affecting anterior tooth display
	Butterfly maxillary permanent central incisors
Alignment	Maxillary diastemata
	Mild mandibular arch perimeter deficiency
Transverse	No deviation
Sagittal	No deviation
Vertical	No deviation

Table 6.6 Enhancement Outcome

Primary Characteristic	Specific Variation	Enhancement
Dentofacial appearance	Unattractive anterior tooth display (diastema, butterfly incisors)	Anterior tooth display improved through diastema closure and tooth alignment
Alignment	Diastema between teeth No. 8 and No. 9	Closed diastema between teeth No. 8 and No. 9
	Crowding teeth No. 22 through No. 27	Aligned teeth No. 22 through No. 27

Case Study 6.3

See Figures 6.13 through 6.17 and Table 6.7.

Orthogonal Analysis

See Table 6.8.

Problem List (Rank Ordered by Patient Preferences)

Maxillary diastemata
Hypertrophied maxillary labial frenum
Anterior tooth size discrepancy (maxillary incisors)
Mild mandibular anterior spacing

Treatment Options

1. Level and align maxillary and mandibular arches
   Redistribute space distal to the maxillary permanent canines
   Frenectomy
2. Level and align maxillary and mandibular arches
   Readjust space in maxillary arch
   Close space in mandibular arch
   Frenectomy
   Cosmetic bonding, teeth No. 7, 8, 9, and 10
3. Level and align maxillary arch
   Readjust space in maxillary arch
   Frenectomy
   Cosmetic bonding, teeth No. 7, 8, 9, and 10
4. No treatment

Unified Final Treatment Plan

Level and align maxillary arch
Readjust space in maxillary arch
Frenectomy

Cosmetic bonding, teeth No. 7, 8, 9, and 10

Therapy

Modified straight wire appliance
Direct bond ↑ limited fixed appliance (2 × 6, canine-to-canine and first molars)
Successive leveling archwires
Working movement (open coil spring and closed coil spring to readjust space)
Frenectomy
Cosmetic bonding, teeth No. 7, 8, 9, and 10

Actual Treatment Time

8 months

Retention

Prebonding

Modified maxillary Hawley retainer with spurs mesial and distal to teeth No. 7, 8, 9, and 10

Postbonding

Maxillary full coverage clear thermoplastic retainer

Enhancement Outcome

See Table 6.9.

Commentary

This patient's chief concern was related to variation in several dentofacial traits composing anterior tooth display. He was pri-
Continued

marily concerned with the "gaps" between his upper front teeth and was not necessarily concerned with the shape or color of the front teeth. A diagnostic setup was performed to simulate: (1) redistribution of space distal to the maxillary canines and (2) redistribution of space between the incisors, followed by cosmetic bonding of all four teeth. The patient was presented with the various treatment alternatives as well as the risks and benefits of each option. Because the patient had a complex smile style and a broad smile aperture, the option of leaving space distal to the maxillary canines was ruled out from an appearance standpoint. The patient selected the option of limited treatment of the maxillary spacing with a combination of orthodontics, frenectomy, and cosmetic bonding. The patient recently completed the cosmetic dental treatment and will be offered the option of gingival recontouring with a soft-tissue diode laser in the future (Swick and Richter 2003) (Fig. 6.18).

Table 6.7 Patient Data

Age	15 Years
Chief complaint	"Gaps between front teeth"
Medical history	Noncontributory
Dental history	Oral hygiene within normal limits
	Low caries rate
	Dental visits at 6-month intervals

Table 6.8 Orthognal Analysis

Dentofacial appearance	Prominent maxillary diastemata negatively affecting anterior tooth display
Alignment	Anterior tooth size discrepancy (narrow maxillary permanent incisors, teeth No. 7, No. 8, No. 9, and No. 10)
	Maxillary diastemata
	Mild mandibular anterior spacing
	Hypertrophied maxillary labial frenum
Transverse	No deviation
Sagittal	No deviation
Vertical	No deviation

Table 6.9 Enhancement Outcome

Primary Characteristic	Specific Variation	Enhancement
Dentofacial appearance	Unattractive anterior tooth display (tooth size, diastemata)	Improved anterior tooth display through tooth movement and cosmetic dentistry
Alignment	Anterior tooth size discrepancy teeth No. 7 through No. 10	Cosmetic bonding teeth No. 7 through No. 10
	Spacing between teeth No. 7 through No. 10	Cosmetic bonding teeth No. 7 through No. 10
	Hypertrophied maxillary labial frenum	Hypertrophied maxillary labial frenum resected

PSYCHOSOCIAL AND PHYSICAL GROWTH STATUS

Chief Concern: *GAPS BETWEEN FRONT TEETH*

Reason for seeking orthodontic advice:

[X] Information
[?] Treatment at this time
[ ] Clarification of previously received information or conflicting information
[ ] Continuation of treatment

Figure 6.13 The patient's chief concern and reason for seeking orthodontic advice.

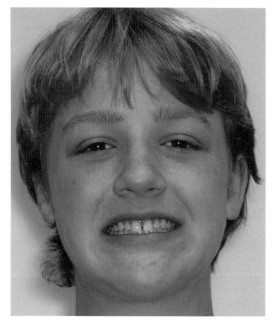

Figure 6.14 Facial view during social smile.

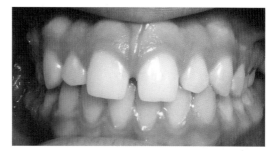

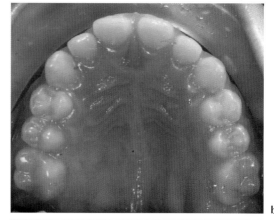

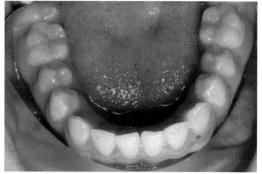

Figure 6.15 (**A**) Front occlusal view. Note the hypertrophied maxillary labial frenum. (**B**) Maxillary occlusal view. (**C**) Mandibular occlusal view.

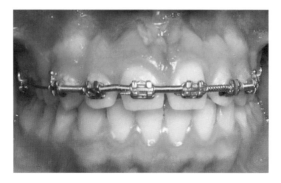

Figure 6.16 Maxillary limited fixed appliance in place. A combination of open coil spring and closed coil spring was used to redistribute space between teeth No. 7 through No. 10, prior to cosmetic bonding. The frenectomy was performed several weeks prior to this visit. Note the excellent tissue healing in this area. (Frenectomy: Dr. Tom Seibert.)

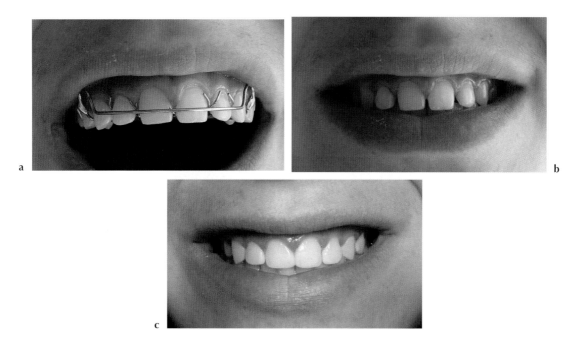

Figure 6.17 (**A**) The maxillary limited fixed appliance was debonded, and a modified maxillary Hawley retainer with spurs mesial and distal to teeth No. 7 through No. 10 was prescribed to the patient for full-time wear until the cosmetic bonding occurred. (**B**) The patient's cropped social smile prior to cosmetic bonding. (**C**) The patient's cropped social smile after cosmetic bonding was completed. (Cosmetic bonding: Dr. Robin Harshaw.)

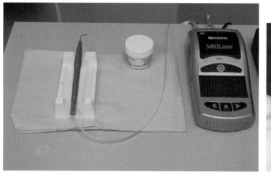
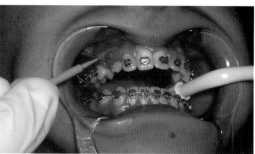

a   b

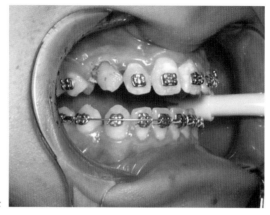

c

Figure 6.18 (**A**) A 980-nanometer (nm) diode laser (SIROLaser, Sirona Dental Systems LLC, Charlotte, North Carolina). The 980-nm wavelength laser has an absorption peak in the water absorption spectrum such that it has 8 times higher water absorption than the 810-nm wavelength laser. The increase in water absorption lends itself to a technique using less conductive energy from a hot tip to the use of more radiant energy for ablation. With the high fluence technique (Swick and Richter 2003), which is characterized by higher power (wattage), a pulsed mode, a lightly activated fiber, and water for tissue cooling, the 980-nm laser yields dramatically better results than the 810-nm laser. By virtue of this understanding of photobiology, charring and crust-like coagulation can be virtually eliminated during laser surgery. Maximum controllable vaporization with adequate coagulation is the goal of all laser surgeries. (**B**) Application of topical anesthesia to the gingival tissues. This patient's maxillary right permanent canine (tooth No. 6) was palatally impacted. In the course of moving the crown of tooth No. 6 labially, excess tissue accumulated on the facial aspect. Tissue recontouring was essential for correct bracket positioning on tooth No. 6. (**C**) The excess tissue was ablated. Note the minimal charring around the gingival margin of tooth No. 6 due to use of the high fluence technique with the 980-nm laser.

Case Study 6.4

See Figures 6.19 through 6.24 and Table 6.10.

Orthogonal Analysis

See Table 6.11.

Problem List (Rank Ordered by Patient Preferences)

Maxillary midline diastema
Hypertrophied maxillary labial frenum
Mild mandibular rotations (teeth No. 22 and No. 27)
"End-on" molar relationship, left side

Treatment Options

1. Level and align maxillary and mandibular arches
   Condense maxillary space
   Improve molar relationship, left side
   Maxillary labial frenectomy
   Gingivectomy (maxillary anterior teeth)
2. Level and align maxillary arch
   Condense maxillary spaces
   Maxillary labial frenectomy
   Gingivectomy (maxillary anterior teeth)
3. No treatment

Unified Final Treatment Plan

Level and align maxillary and mandibular arches
Condense maxillary space
Improve molar relationship, left side
Maxillary labial frenectomy
Gingivectomy (maxillary anterior teeth)

Therapy

Modified straight wire appliance
Direct bond ↑↓ fixed appliances (including second molars)
Successive leveling archwires
Working movement (space closure)
Interarch elastics if needed
Frenectomy and gingivectomy

Actual Treatment Time

Nineteen months

Retention

Direct bond palatal wire between tooth No. 8 and tooth No. 9
Maxillary Hawley retainer to be worn at night only
Fixed lingual canine-to-canine retainer

Enhancement Outcome

See Table 6.12.

Commentary

This patient's chief concern was related to variation in several dentofacial traits composing anterior tooth display. In particular, she was unhappy with the maxillary midline diastema, hypertrophied maxillary labial frenum, and hypertrophied gingival contours. The patient was presented with the various treatment alternatives as well as the risks and benefits of each option. The patient's mother articulated a need for occlusal "perfection" and elected full treatment for her daughter.

From an anatomic standpoint, this patient had a thick/flat periodontal biotype, similar to the patient in Case Study 6.2. Space closure during the working movements of orthodontic treatment aggravated the hypertrophied labial frenum and gingival tissues, requiring an "emergency" frenectomy and gingivectomy. The periodontist altered the gingival contours, increasing vertical tooth display and giving the interdental papillae a scalloped look. As in Case Study 6.2, it was recommended that the fixed palatal wire between tooth No. 8 and tooth No. 9 remain in place for an indefinite period of time.

Table 6.10 Patient Data

Age	11 Years, 11 months
Chief complaint	"She wants straight teeth and no space in front, a better smile"
Medical history	Noncontributory
Dental history	Oral hygiene within normal limits
	Low caries rate
	Dental visits at 6-month intervals
	Laser frenectomy (maxillary labial and mandibular lingual)

Table 6.11 Orthognal Analysis

Dentofacial appearance	Prominent maxillary midline diastema negatively affecting anterior tooth display
Alignment	Maxillary midline diastema
	Mild mandibular rotations (teeth No. 22 and No. 27)
Transverse	No deviation
Sagittal	"End-on" molar relationship, left side
Vertical	No deviation

Table 6.12 Enhancement Outcome

Primary Characteristic	Specific Variation	Enhancement
Dentofacial appearance	Unattractive anterior tooth display (diastema, gingival contours)	Closed diastema between teeth No. 8 and No. 9
		Gingivectomy improved gingival display
Alignment	Diastema between teeth No. 8 and No. 9	Closed diastema between teeth No. 8 and No. 9
	Rotations	Derotated teeth No. 22 and No. 27
	Hypertrophied maxillary labial frenum	Hypertrophied maxillary labial frenum resected
Sagittal	"End-on" molar relationship left side	Corrected left molar relationship

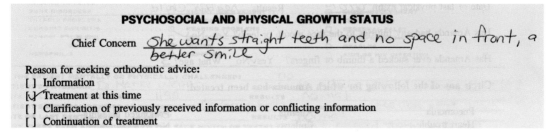

PSYCHOSOCIAL AND PHYSICAL GROWTH STATUS

Chief Concern _She wants straight teeth and no space in front, a better smile_

Reason for seeking orthodontic advice:
[ ] Information
[✓] Treatment at this time
[ ] Clarification of previously received information or conflicting information
[ ] Continuation of treatment

Figure 6.19 The patient's chief concern and reason for seeking orthodontic advice.

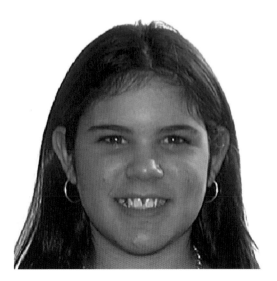

Figure 6.20 Facial view during social smile.

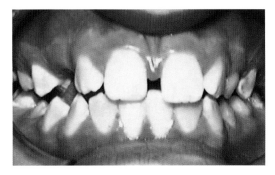

Figure 6.21 Front occlusal view. Note the hypertrophied maxillary labial frenum.

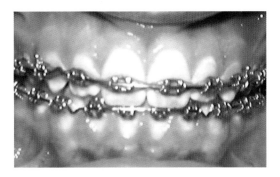

Figure 6.22 Maxillary and mandibular fixed appliances at the completion of treatment. In the course of the working movement (space closure), the patient developed significant gingival hypertrophy. This photograph was taken several weeks after the maxillary labial frenectomy and gingivectomy. (Peridontist: Dr. Cyril Evian.)

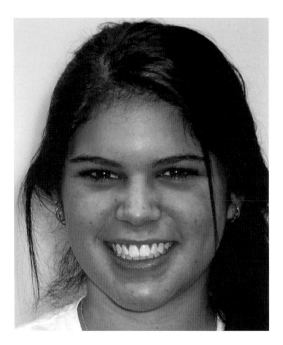

Figure 6.23 Post-treatment facial view during social smile.

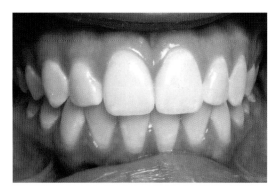

Figure 6.24 Post-treatment front occlusal view.

See Figures 6.25 through 6.30 and Table 6.13.

Orthogonal Analysis

See Table 6.14.

Problem List (Rank Ordered by Patient Preferences)

Maxillary diastemata
Moderate maxillary arch perimeter deficiency
Moderate mandibular arch perimeter deficiency
Anterior deep bite

Treatment Options

1. Extract maxillary and mandibular first premolars
   Level and align maxillary and mandibular arches
   Condense remaining spaces
   Improve overbite
2. Level and align maxillary and mandibular arches
   Condense maxillary anterior spaces
   Create space for maxillary and mandibular permanent canines (teeth No. 6, 11, 22, and 27)
   Improve overbite
3. No treatment

Unified Final Treatment Plan

Therapeutic Diagnosis

Level and align maxillary and mandibular arches
Condense maxillary anterior space
Create additional space for maxillary and mandibular permanent canines (teeth No. 6, 11, 22, and 27)
Improve overbite

Therapy

Modified straight wire appliance
Direct bond ↑↓ fixed appliances (including second molars)
Successive leveling archwires (bite opening)
Working movement (condense space in maxillary arch via elastomeric thread and space gaining in both arches via compressed coil springs)
Interarch elastics if needed

Actual Treatment Time

Thirty months

Retention

Direct bond palatal wire between tooth No. 8 and tooth No. 9
Maxillary Hawley retainer to be worn at night only
Fixed lingual canine-to-canine retainer

Enhancement Outcome

See Table 6.15.

Commentary

This patient's chief concern was related to anterior tooth display. Specifically, the patient and parent were dissatisfied with the maxillary anterior diastemata. Clinical
Continued

examination and diagnostic imaging revealed a moderate arch perimeter deficiency in both arches. At the doctor–patient conference, the parent and patient were apprised of the extent of crowding and made aware that treatment may require the extraction of permanent teeth. Both a nonextraction (therapeutic diagnosis) approach and a four-premolar extraction approach were presented to them. The patient's mother was absolutely opposed to extraction, which ruled out that approach. Thus, a nonextraction approach was undertaken, the tentative diagnosis of "moderate" arch perimeter deficiency was confirmed, and the treatment goals were ultimately achieved. Although the nonextraction treatment created slightly greater facial convexity and a fuller profile, the patient's overall dentofacial appearance was improved.

However, at the completion of active treatment, the patient's mother began to recriminate about the nonextraction decision. She became concerned whether any "long-term" harm had been done to her daughter's facial balance. Diagnostic images were taken, and a doctor–patient conference was scheduled. After reviewing the post-treatment imaging and comparing it to the pretreatment database, all parties agreed that a mild increase in facial convexity and tooth angulation had occurred but was acceptable from a dentofacial appearance standpoint. Five years later, the mother asked if her daughter could be reevaluated along the same lines. New images were taken, and facial analysis determined that the profile had become less convex than at the completion of active treatment. This further confirmed that the original nonextraction decision was indeed the correct one in this case.

Table 6.13 Patient Data

Age	9 Years, 5 months
Chief complaint	"Crowding, small oral cavity"
Medical history	Eye surgery to correct exotropia
Dental history	Oral hygiene within normal limits
	Low caries rate
	Dental visits at 6-month intervals

Table 6.14 Orthognal Analysis

Dentofacial appearance	Maxillary diastemata negatively affecting anterior tooth display
Alignment	Moderate maxillary arch perimeter deficiency
	Moderate mandibular arch perimeter deficiency
Transverse	No deviation
Sagittal	No deviation
Vertical	Anterior deep bite (dental)

Table 6.15 Enhancement Outcome

Primary Characteristic	Specific Variation	Enhancement
Dentofacial appearance	Unatttractive anterior tooth display (diastemata)	Improved anterior tooth display through diastemata closure
Alignment	Arch perimeter deficiency (maxillary and mandibular arches)	Created space for permanent canines and aligned both arches
Vertical	Dental deep bite	Bite opening mechanics improved overbite

HAS EITHER PARENT HAD ORTHODONTIC TREATMENT?   YES ☐ NO ☑
CHIEF CONCERN OF ~~PATIENT~~: *PARENT — CROWDING, SMALL ORAL CAVITY*

Figure 6.25 The patient's chief concern and reason for seeking orthodontic advice.

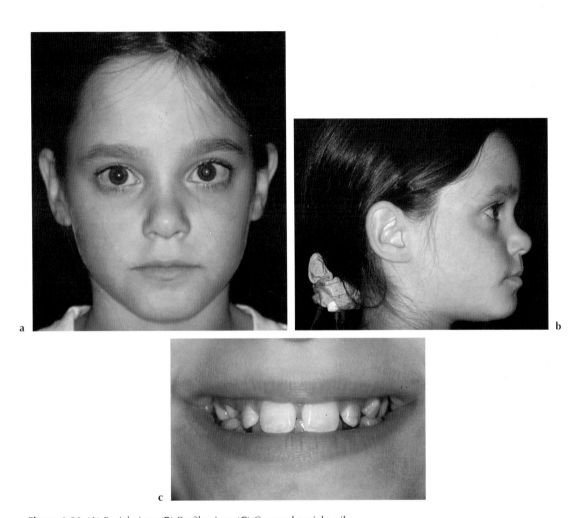

Figure 6.26 (**A**) Facial view. (**B**) Profile view. (**C**) Cropped social smile.

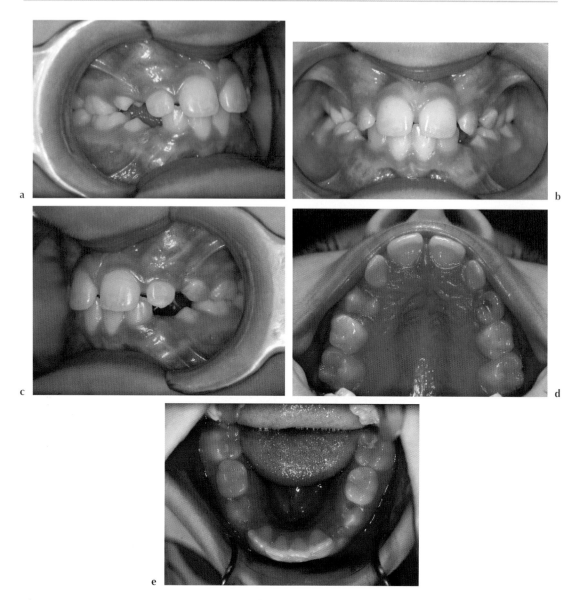

Figure 6.27 (**A–E**) Occlusal views.

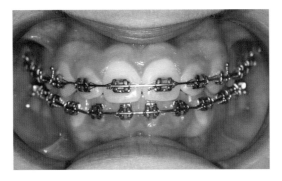

Figure 6.28 Maxillary and mandibular fixed appliances at the completion of treatment.

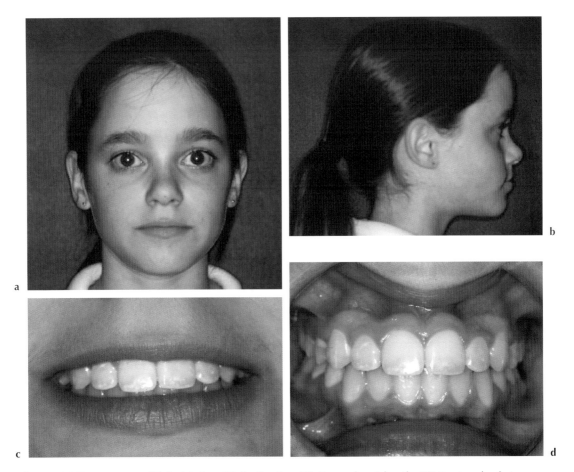

Figure 6.29 Post-treatment. (**A**) Facial view. (**B**) Profile view. (**C**) Cropped social smile. (**D**) Front occlusal view.

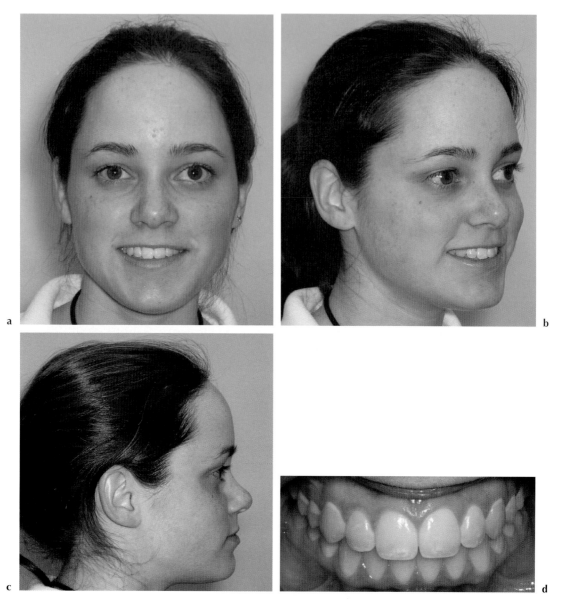

Figure 6.30 Five years post-treatment. (**A**) Facial view during social smile. (**B**) Three-quarter facial view during social smile. (**C**) Profile view. (**D**) Front occlusal view.

Case Study 6.6

See Figures 6.31 through 6.36 and Table 6.16.

Orthogonal Analysis

See Table 6.17.

Problem List (Rank Ordered by Patient Preferences)

Severe maxillary arch perimeter deficiency
Severe mandibular arch perimeter deficiency
Three of four permanent canines "blocked out" of arches
Moderately retroclined maxillary incisors
Anterior deep bite (skeletal and dental)
Excessive gingival display during smile

Treatment Options

1. Extract four first premolars
   Reevaluate when all permanent teeth emerge
2. Attempt a nonextraction approach
   Level and align maxillary and mandibular arches
   Create space for "blocked out" permanent canines
   Improve overbite/overjet relationship
   Improve gingival display via intrusion and/or clinical crown lengthening
3. No treatment

Unified Final Treatment Plan

Extract four first premolars
Reevaluate when all permanent teeth emerge for:

Level and align maxillary and mandibular arches

Condense remaining extraction spaces
Improve overbite/overjet relationship
Improve angulation of maxillary incisors
Improve gingival display via intrusion and/or clinical crown lengthening

Therapy

Modified straight wire appliance
Direct bond ⇅ fixed appliances (including second molars)
Successive leveling archwires (bite opening)
Working movements (space condensing in maxillary and mandibular arches, labial crown torque in maxillary incisors)
Interarch elastics if needed

Actual Treatment Time

Twenty-two months

Retention

Maxillary Hawley retainer with a continuous labial bow and Adams clasps on the first permanent molars and an anterior bite plane
Mandibular Hawley retainer with continuous labial bow and Adams clasps on the first permanent molars

Enhancement Outcome

See Table 6.18.

Commentary

Many authors have espoused modification of dentofacial traits with nonextraction treatment as the preferred approach in con-

Continued

temporary orthodontics. However, there are some variations in dentofacial traits (e.g., severe arch perimeter deficiency and recognizable dental compensation for an underlying skeletal discrepancy) that require the extraction of permanent teeth. The decision to extract in orthodontics is based on the fact that the ability of the soft tissues to adapt to changes in tooth-jaw relationships is far narrower than the anatomic boundaries in modifying occlusal relationships (Ackerman and Proffit 1997). For example, it is not unusual to reduce overjet in a growing patient by 7 to 10 mm. However, the tolerances for soft-tissue adaptation from equilibrium, periodontal, tempormandibular joint, and facial balance perspectives are in the range of 2 to 3 mm for lower arch expansion and even less for condylar position. In summary, it is the ability of the soft tissues to adapt to changes in tooth or jaw positions that determines therapeutic modifiability in orthodontic treatment.

This patient's parents sought a second orthodontic opinion to investigate the possibility of nonextraction treatment. In reviewing the clinical database, the other orthodontist thought that extraction treatment might overretract the incisors and "flatten" the patient's profile. An evaluation of the progress imaging taken after extraction of the four first premolars demonstrated very little residual space after the eruption of the permanent canines. The orthodontic mechanotherapy that was ultimately used applied minimal anchorage, which translated to minimal retraction of the incisors.

This patient's severe arch perimeter deficiency would have required dental arch expansion beyond the limits of soft tissue adaptation. Consequently, there would have been negative repercussions on dentofacial appearance and stability. The extraction of four first premolars was imperative for enhancement of this patient's dentofacial appearance.

PSYCHOSOCIAL AND PHYSICAL GROWTH STATUS

Chief Concern _____

Reason for seeking orthodontic advice:
[ ] Information
—[ ] Treatment at this time
[ ] Clarification of previously received information or conflicting information
[ ]˙ Continuation of treatment

Figure 6.31 The patient's chief concern and reason for seeking orthodontic advice.

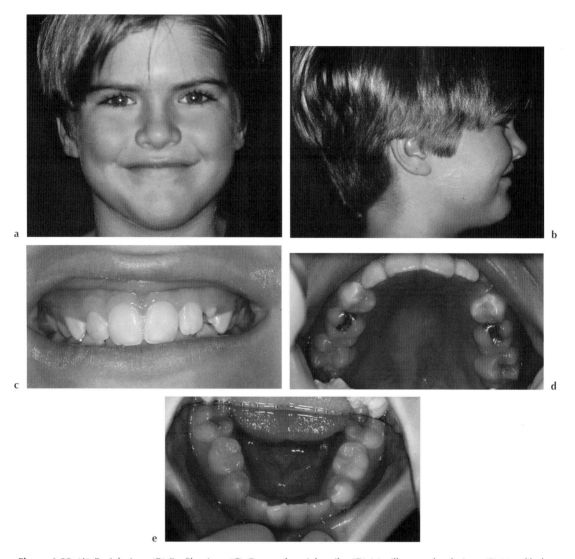

Figure 6.32 (**A**) Facial view. (**B**) Profile view. (**C**) Cropped social smile. (**D**) Maxillary occlusal view. (**E**) Mandibular occlusal view.

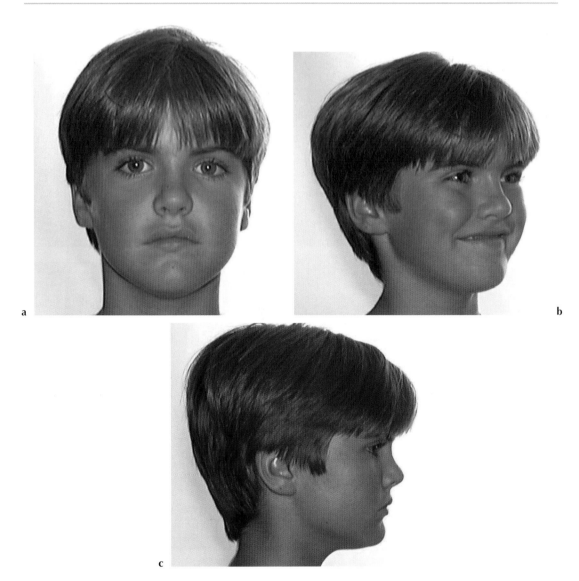

Figure 6.33 Postextraction of maxillary and mandibular first premolars, images taken 1 year after the original examination. (**A**) Facial view. (**B**) Three-quarter facial view during social smile. (**C**) Profile view.

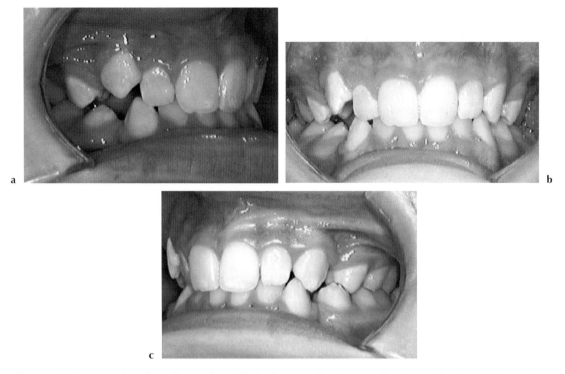

Figure 6.34 Postextraction of maxillary and mandibular first premolars, images taken 1 year after the original examination. (**A**–**C**) Occlusal views.

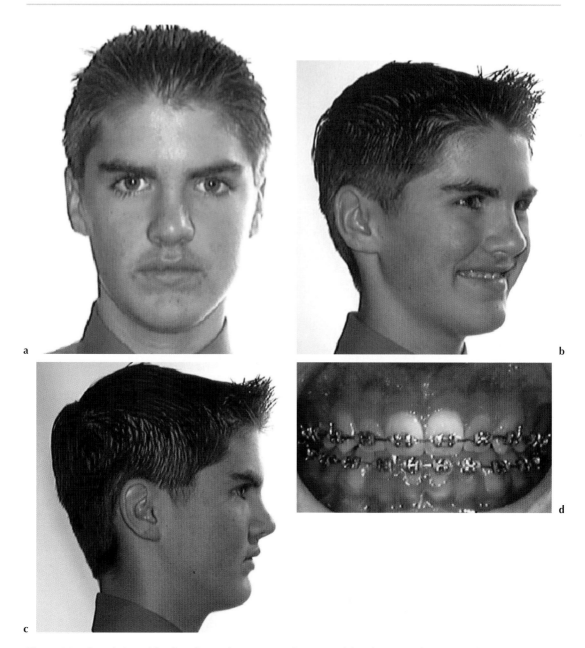

Figure 6.35 Completion of fixed appliance therapy, 1 week prior to debond. (**A**) Facial view. (**B**) Three-quarter facial view during social smile. (**C**) Profile view. (**D**) Front occlusal view.

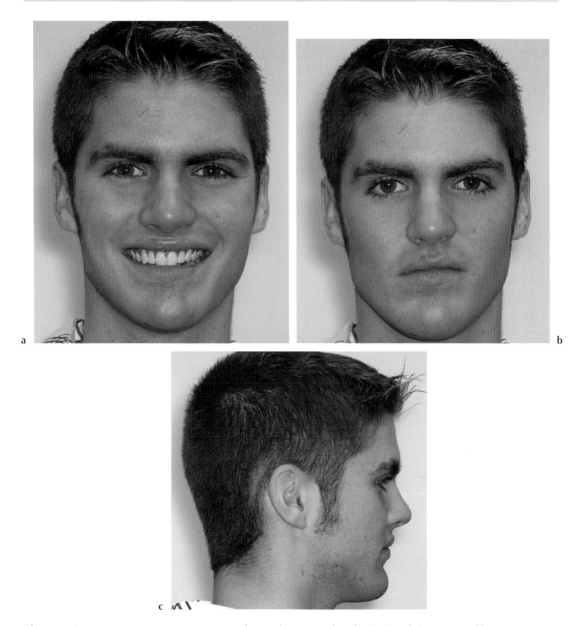

Figure 6.36 Five years post-treatment. (**A**) Facial view during social smile. (**B**) Facial view. (**C**) Profile view.

Table 6.16 Patient Data

Age	10 Years, 11 months
Chief complaint	The parent and patient did not indicate a chief concern on the health questionnaire. In the course of the doctor–patient interview, it became clear that the parents were seeking orthodontic advice on the recommendation of the dentist. His concern was the maxillary and mandibular arch perimeter deficiencies.
Medical history	Noncontributory
Dental history	Oral hygiene within normal limits
	Low caries rate
	Dental visits at 6-month intervals

Table 6.17 Orthognal Analysis

Dentofacial appearance	Excessive gingival display during smile
Alignment	Severe maxillary arch perimeter deficiency
	Severe mandibular arch perimeter deficiency
	Three of four permanent canines "blocked out" of arches
	Moderately retroclined maxillary incisors
Transverse	No deviation
Sagittal	No deviation
Vertical	Anterior deep bite (skeletal and dental)

Table 6.18 Enhancement Outcome

Primary Characteristic	Specific Variation	Enhancement
Dentofacial appearance	Unattractive anterior tooth display (excessive gingival display)	Anterior tooth display improved by reducing gingival display
Alignment	Arch perimeter deficiency (maxillary and mandibular arches) Incisor Inclination	Extracted teeth and aligned arches Labial crown torque improved maxillary incisor angulation
Vertical	Anterior deep bite (dental and skeletal)	Bite opening mechanics improved overbite and gingival display

Case Study 6.7

See Figures 6.37 through 6.41 and Table 6.19.

Orthogonal Analysis

See Table 6.20.

Problem List (Rank Ordered by Patient Preferences)

Midface deficiency
Anteriorly divergent profile
Excessive gingival display
Mandibular arch perimeter deficiency
Class III skeletal and dental (maxillary retrusion)
Edge-to-edge anterior bite/shallow overbite

Treatment Options

1. Surgical orthodontics:
   Level and align maxillary and mandibular arches
   Decompensate mandibular incisors
   Le Fort I maxillary osteotomy with maxillary advancement and anterior vertical shortening
2. No treatment

Unified Final Treatment Plan

Surgical orthodontics:
Level and align maxillary and mandibular arches
Decompensate mandibular incisors
Le Fort I maxillary osteotomy with maxillary advancement and anterior vertical shortening

Therapy

Surgical straight wire appliance
Band all first and second permanent molars
Direct bond ↑↓ fixed appliances on the remaining teeth
Successive leveling archwires
Class II elastics to decompensate mandibular incisors
Finishing elastics

Actual Treatment Time

Nineteen months

Retention

Direct bond palatal wire between tooth No. 8 and tooth No. 9
Maxillary Hawley retainer to be worn at night only
Fixed lingual canine-to-canine retainer bonded to each tooth (teeth No. 22 to No. 27)

Enhancement Outcome

See Table 6.21.

Commentary

This patient's chief concern was her dentofacial appearance. She exhibited a clinical maxillary deficiency characterized by a lack of skeletal support for the soft tissues of the infraorbital, paranasal, and upper lip regions. The patient was an excellent candidate for maxillary advancement surgery

Continued

because of the appearance of her midface morphology. Surgical correction involved maxillary advancement at the Le Fort I level (6 mm) and maxillary anterior vertical shortening (2 mm).

The surgical orthodontic treatment for this patient was based on facial skeletal expansion (Rosen 1992). Facial skeletal expansion is delineated by two important concepts. The first concept is that facial proportions and dimensions beyond those, which are considered normal, may be extremely attractive in a given individual. The second concept is that the soft-tissue response to skeletal expansion is more favorable and predictable than it is to skel-etal contraction in providing for well-supported soft tissues. In this particular case, maxillary advancement was used to improve the appearance of the midface by enlarging the skeletal scaffold. Mandibular setback surgery, if used in this case, would have only diminished chin projection and not addressed the nature of the appearance problem, that is, maxillary hypoplasia anteroposteriorly.

In practice, surgical orthodontic planning should be predicated on clinical examination of the patient and not normative data taken from unscientific cephalometric standards.

Table 6.19 Patient Data

Age	16 Years, 1 month
Chief complaint	"Alignment of jaw/arrangement of lower teeth"
Medical history	Acne, takes Accutane 60 mg
Dental history	Mild marginal gingivitis
	Low caries rate
	Dental visits at 6-month intervals

Table 6.20 Orthognal Analysis

Dentofacial appearance	Midface deficiency (maxillary hypoplasia, anteroposteriorly)
	Anteriorly divergent profile
	Short philtrum height
	Excessive gingival display
Alignment	Mandibular arch perimeter deficiency
	Retroclined mandibular incisors (dental compensation for Class III skeletal pattern)
	Mild maxillary spacing
Transverse	No deviation
Sagittal	Class III skeletal and dental (maxillary hypoplasia)
Vertical	Edge-to-edge anterior bite/shallow overbite

Table 6.21 Enhancement Outcome

Primary Characteristic	Specific Variation	Enhancement
Dentofacial appearance	Midface deficiency Anterior divergence Unattractive anterior tooth display (excessive gingival display)	Maxillary advancement surgery corrected midface deficiency Maxillary advancement surgery eliminated anterior divergence Maxillary impaction reduced gingival display
Alignment	Arch perimeter deficiency (mandibular arch)	Aligned mandibular arch
Sagittal	Maxillary hypoplasia	Maxillary advancement surgery improved position of maxilla
Vertical	Edge-to-edge anterior bite/shallow overbite	Maxillary surgical movement corrected overbite

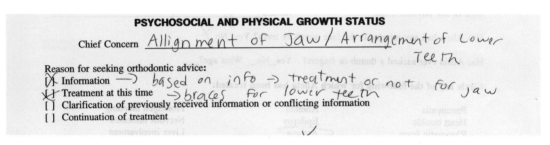

Figure 6.37 The patient's chief concern and reason for seeking orthodontic advice.

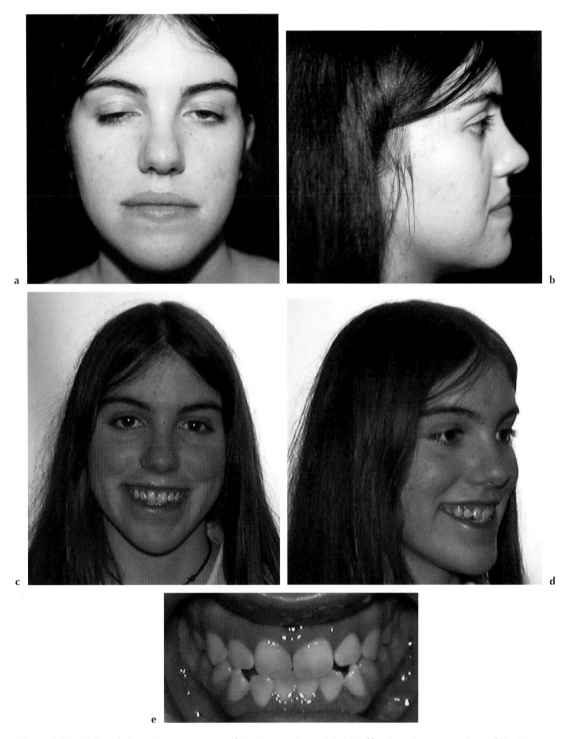

Figure 6.38 (**A**) Facial view. (Image courtesy of Dr. Harvey Rosen.) (**B**) Profile view. (Image courtesy of Dr. Harvey Rosen.) (**C**) Facial view during social smile. (**D**) Three-quarter facial view during social smile. (**E**) Front occlusal view.

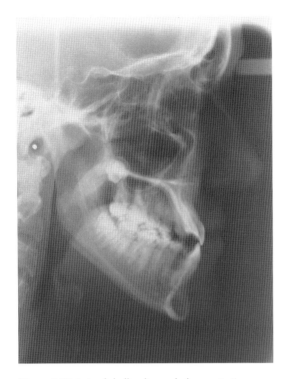

Figure 6.39 Lateral skull radiograph demonstrating maxillary hypoplasia anteroposteriorly.

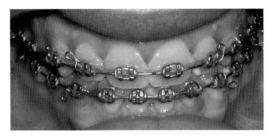

Figure 6.40 Orthodontic finishing postsurgery. Kobayashi hooks on the anterior brackets serve as attachment points for elastics worn in a rectangular "box" pattern.

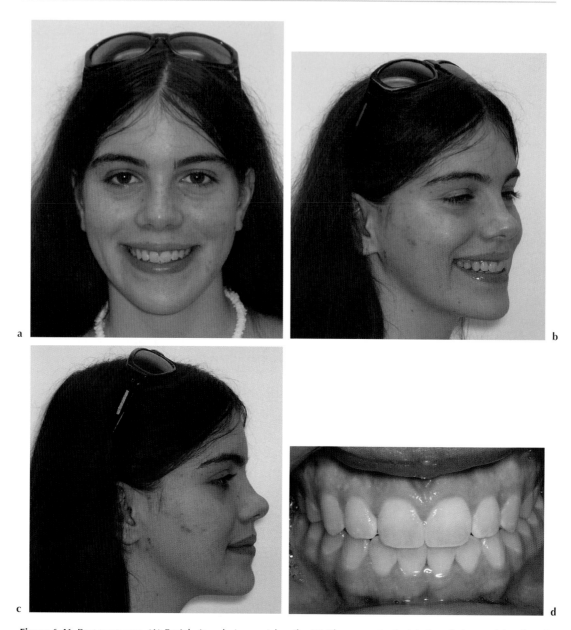

a   b

c   d

Figure 6.41 Post-treatment. (**A**) Facial view during social smile. (**B**) Three-quarter facial view during social smile. (**C**) Profile view. (**D**) Front occlusal view. (Orthognathic surgery: Dr. Harvey Rosen.)

Case Study 6.8

See Figures 6.42 through 6.46 and Table 6.22.

Orthogonal Analysis

See Table 6.23.

Problem List (Rank Ordered by Patient Preferences)

Chin form and projection
Vertical maxillary excess (VME)
Lip incompetence
Excessive gingival display during enjoyment smile
Maxillary and mandibular arch perimeter deficiencies
Class II molar relationship

Treatment Options

1. Remove chin implant and cheek implants
   Surgical orthodontics:
   Level and align maxillary and mandibular arches
   Le Fort I maxillary osteotomy with maxillary impaction (4 mm)
   Autorotation of the mandible to gain chin projection and placement of new chin implant
2. No treatment

Unified Final Treatment Plan

Remove chin implant and cheek implants
Surgical orthodontics:

Level and align maxillary and mandibular arches

Le Fort I maxillary osteotomy with maxillary impaction (4 mm)
Autorotation of the mandible to gain chin projection
Placement of new chin implant

Therapy

Surgical straight wire appliance
Band all first and second permanent molars
Direct bond ↑↓ fixed appliances on the remaining teeth
Successive leveling archwires
Finishing elastics

Actual Treatment Time

Eleven months

Retention

Direct bond palatal wire between tooth No. 8 and tooth No. 9
Maxillary Hawley retainer to be worn at night only
Fixed lingual canine-to-canine retainer bonded to each tooth (teeth No. 22 to No. 27)

Enhancement Outcome

See Table 6.24.

Commentary

At age 25, this patient underwent an "extreme makeover" of dentofacial appearance. A plastic and reconstructive surgeon

Continued

placed Proplast (Vitek) implants in the cheeks and gonial angles, as well as performing a genioplasty. A decade later, the patient was still dissatisfied with her chin projection and the surgeon placed a Proplast implant in the chin. All of these procedures were an attempt to camouflage the patient's insufficient skeletal support of the mid and lower face. The morphologic features of vertical maxillary excess were never addressed in his therapeutic plan. After suffering the combined effects of facial aging and a poorly conceived facial plastic surgical plan, this patient decided to revisit enhancement of her dentofacial appearance.

The proposed retreatment entailed a combination of orthodontics and orthognathic surgery. Presurgical orthodontics involved (1) leveling and aligning both arches and (2) reestablishing coordinated catenary arch forms. Surgical removal of the old chin implant was performed during the presurgical orthodontic treatment. It was decided that mandibular advancement surgery was too risky due to the poor quality of bone (a result of the gonial angle implants) in the region where the sagittal split osteotomy would have to be made. The final surgical plan was a Le Fort I maxillary osteotomy with impaction to shorten lower facial height, improve gingival display, and autorotate the mandible creating more chin projection. The cheek implants were removed during surgery, and a new chin implant was placed to give additional support to the soft-tissue chin.

Table 6.22 Patient Data

Age	40 Years, 3 months
Chief complaint	This patient did not indicate a chief concern on the health questionnaire. She was referred for an orthodontic consultation by a plastic and reconstructive surgeon in anticipation of surgical-orthodontic treatment.
Medical history	Proplast cheek implants
	Proplast gonial angle implants
	Genioplasty followed by a Proplast chin implant 10 years later
	Right knee anterior cruciate ligament (ACL) reconstruction
	Benign ovarian tumor removed
Dental history	Orthodontic treatment as an adolescent (four premolar extraction)
	Third molar removal
	Restorative dentistry (caries in posterior teeth)
	Generalized horizontal bone loss, no active periodontal disease
	Dental visits at 6-month intervals

Table 6.23 Orthognal Analysis

Dentofacial appearance	Vertical maxillary excess (VME)
	Lip incompetence (everted lower lip)
	Deepened sublabial furrow
	Unattractive chin form
	Inadequate chin projection
	Excessive gingival display during enjoyment smile
Alignment	Maxillary arch perimeter deficiency
	Mandibular arch perimeter deficiency
Transverse	No deviation
Sagittal	Class II, division I skeletal and dental (mandibular retrognathia)
Vertical	Vertical maxillary excess (VME)

Table 6.24 Enhancement Outcome

Primary Characteristic	Specific Variation	Enhancement
Dentofacial appearance	Vertical maxillary excess (VME) Unattractive chin form and projection Unattractive anterior tooth display (excessive gingival display)	Maxillary impaction surgery reduced VME Placement of new chin implant and autorotation of the mandible improved chin form and projection Maxillary impaction surgery reduced gingival display
Alignment	Arch perimeter deficiency (maxillary and mandibular arches)	Aligned both arches
Sagittal	Mandibular retrognathia/chin projection	Improved via autorotation and placement of new chin implant
Vertical	VME	Maxillary impaction reduced vertical length of lower facial third

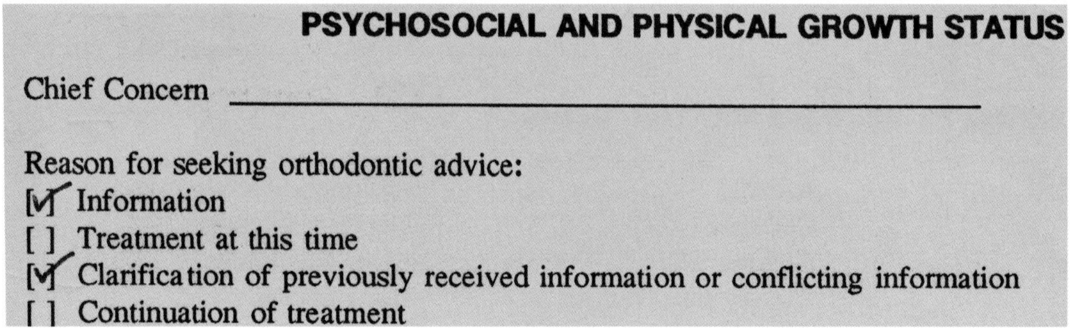

PSYCHOSOCIAL AND PHYSICAL GROWTH STATUS

Chief Concern _____

Reason for seeking orthodontic advice:
[✓] Information
[ ] Treatment at this time
[✓] Clarification of previously received information or conflicting information
[ ] Continuation of treatment

Figure 6.42 The patient's chief concern and reason for seeking orthodontic advice.

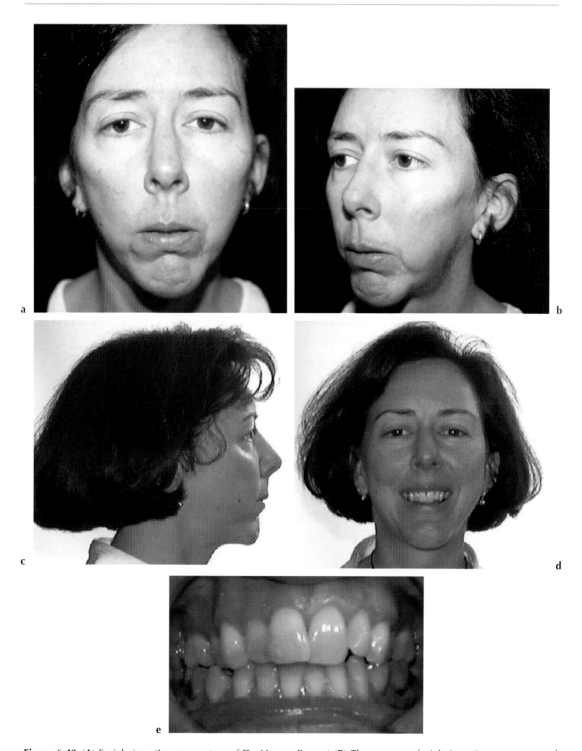

Figure 6.43 (**A**) Facial view. (Image courtesy of Dr. Harvey Rosen.) (**B**) Three-quarter facial view. (Image courtesy of Dr. Harvey Rosen.) (**C**) Profile view. (**D**) Facial view during social smile. The excessive gingival display was seen during the transition from social smile to enjoyment smile. (**E**) Front occlusal view.

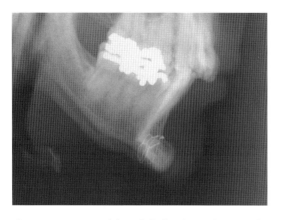

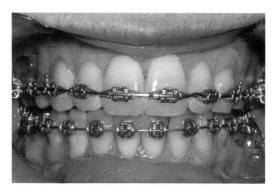

Figure 6.45 Fixed appliances during orthodontic finishing postsurgery.

Figure 6.44 Cropped lateral skull radiograph. Note the suspensory wires securing the patients unattractive chin implant to the anterior portion of the mandible.

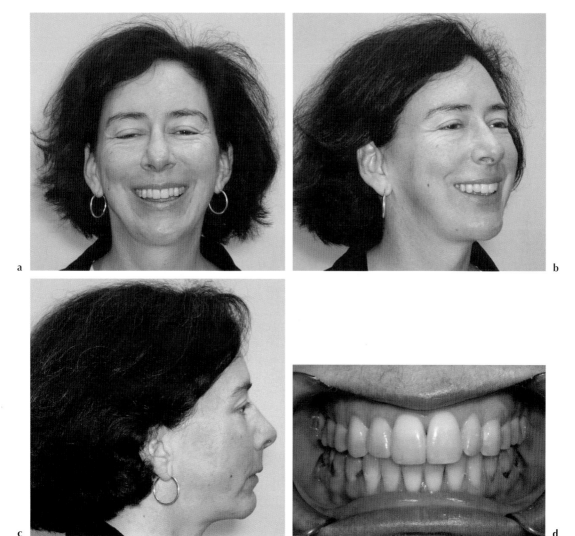

Figure 6.46 Post-treatment. (**A**) Facial view during social smile. (**B**) Three-quarter facial view during social smile. (**C**) Profile view. (**D**) Front occlusal view. (Orthognathic surgery: Dr. Harvey Rosen.)

Case Study 6.9

See Figures 6.47 through 6.49 and Table 6.25.

Orthogonal Analysis

See Table 6.26.

Problem List (Rank Ordered by Patient Preferences)

Roll of the esthetic line of the dentition (up to the left side)
Maxillary spacing
Mild mandibular anterior crowding
Shallow overbite

Treatment Options

1. Level and align maxillary arch
   Correct roll of the esthetic line of the dentition
   Condense spaces
   Realign mandibular anterior teeth
   Improve overbite
2. Level and align maxillary arch
   Correct roll of the esthetic line of the dentition
   Condense spaces
   Improve overbite
3. Realign mandibular anterior teeth
4. No treatment

Unified Final Treatment Plan

Level and align maxillary arch
Correct roll of the esthetic line of the dentition
Condense spaces
Realign mandibular anterior teeth
Improve overbite

Therapy

Modified straight wire appliance
Direct bond ↑ fixed appliance (first molar-to–first molar)
Successive leveling archwires
Working movement (elastomeric thread to close space)
Polish off remnants of fixed canine-to-canine retainer
Mandibular removable spring aligner

Actual Treatment Time

Eight months

Retention

Maxillary nightguard
Mandibular removable spring aligner

Enhancement Outcome

See Table 6.27.

Commentary

The patient's chief concern was the spacing of the upper teeth, the roll of the esthetic line of the dentition, and their effect on anterior tooth display. He was originally treated to a successful orthodontic outcome as an adolescent in California. Several years into retention, he stopped wearing his upper retainer. As an adult, he had been wearing a maxillary nightguard to counteract the effects of nocturnal bruxism.

The key to leveling the roll of the esthetic line of the dentition in this case was differential bracketing of the anterior teeth.

The brackets were placed more gingivally beginning with the maxillary left permanent central incisor moving posteriorly to the maxillary left permanent canine. As treatment progressed through successive leveling archwires, the maxillary left permanent central incisor, lateral incisor, and canine were differentially extruded to eliminate the roll effect and improve overbite.

Table 6.25 Patient Data

Age	27 Years, 4 months
Chief complaint	"Cosmetic"
Medical history	Latex allergy
Dental history	Oral hygiene within normal limits
	Low caries rate
	Dental visits at 6-month intervals
	Orthodontic treatment for 2 years as an adolescent
	Third molar removal
	Bruxism, wears a maxillary nightguard
	Broken fixed lingual canine-to-canine retainer bonded to each tooth (teeth No. 22 through No. 27)

Table 6.26 Orthognal Analysis

Dentofacial appearance	Unattractive anterior tooth display
	Roll of the esthetic line of the dentition (up to the left side)
Alignment	Maxillary spacing
	Very mild mandibular anterior crowding
Transverse	No deviation
Sagittal	No deviation
Vertical	Shallow overbite

Table 6.27 Enhancement Outcome

Primary Characteristic	Specific Variation	Enhancement
Dentofacial appearance	Unattractive anterior tooth display (roll of the esthetic line of the dentition up to the left side)	Tooth movement improved the orientation of the esthetic line of the dentition and anterior tooth display
Alignment	Maxillary spacing	Condensed spaces
	Mild mandibular anterior crowding	Realigned mandibular anterior teeth
Vertical	Shallow overbite	Extrusion of incisors improved overbite

PSYCHOSOCIAL AND PHYSICAL GROWTH STATUS

Your Chief Concern: _____Cosmetic_____

Reason for seeking orthodontic advice:

[✓] Information
[ ] Treatment at this time
[ ] Clarification of previously received information or conflicting information
[ ] Continuation of treatment

Figure 6.47 The patient's chief concern and reason for seeking orthodontic advice.

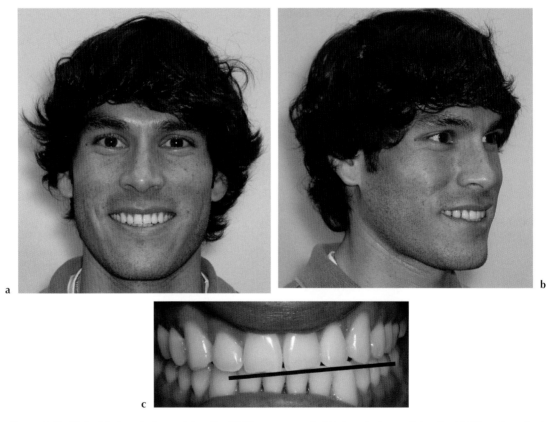

Figure 6.48 (**A**) Facial view during social smile. (**B**) Three-quarter facial view during social smile. (**C**) Note the roll of the esthetic line of the dentition, up to the left side.

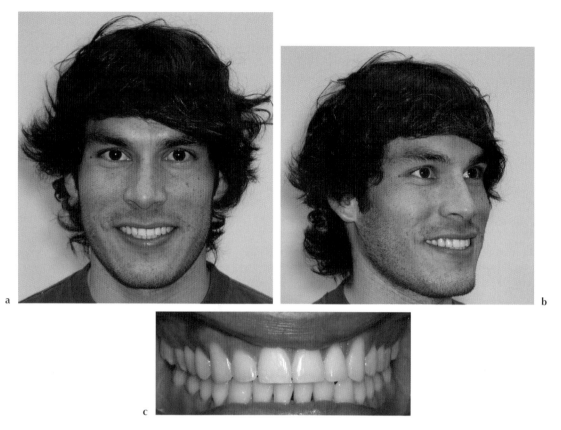

Figure 6.49 Post-treatment. (**A**) Facial view during social smile. (**B**) Three-quarter facial view during social smile. (**C**) Front occlusal view.

Case Study 6.10

See Figures 6.50 through 6.53 and Table 6.28.

Orthogonal Analysis

See Table 6.29.

Problem List (Rank Ordered by Patient Preferences)

Thin/scalloped periodontal biotype
Maxillary left permanent central incisor (tooth No. 9) labioverted and 1 mm longer than the right permanent central incisor (tooth No. 8)
Mild mandibular rotations
Class II molar left side
Anterior deep bite

Treatment Options

1. Level and align maxillary anterior teeth
   Reproximate contact area between teeth No. 8 and No. 9 (lengthen incisoapically and broaden faciolingually)
   Improve anterior tooth display
   Level and align mandibular anterior teeth
   Improve molar relationship
   Improve overbite
2. Level and align maxillary anterior teeth
   Reproximate contact area between teeth No. 8 and No. 9 (lengthen incisoapically and broaden faciolingually)
   Improve anterior tooth display
3. No treatment

Unified Final Treatment Plan

Level and align maxillary anterior teeth
Reproximate contact area between teeth No. 8 and No. 9 (lengthen incisoapically and broaden faciolingually)
Improve anterior tooth display

Therapy

Modified straight wire appliance
Direct bond ↑ limited fixed appliance (2 × 4, lateral–to–lateral and first molars)
Successive leveling archwires
Reproximate contact area between teeth No. 8 and No. 9

Actual Treatment Time

Four months

Retention

Direct bond palatal wire between tooth No. 8 and tooth No. 9
Maxillary Hawley retainer to be worn at night only

Enhancement Outcome

See Table 6.30.

Commentary

This patient's chief concern was unattractive anterior tooth display related to the maxillary left permanent central incisor (tooth No. 9) being labioverted and 1 mm longer than the maxillary right permanent central incisor (tooth No. 8). She was originally treated to a successful orthodontic outcome as an adolescent in Virginia. The patient had stopped wearing her maxillary retainer several years into retention and recently noticed changes in anterior tooth display.

Orthodontic retreatment in this patient's case was complicated by the sequelae of the thin/scalloped periodontal biotype. Unattractive "black triangles" already existed in the mandibular anterior interdental spaces, and the likelihood that this patient would develop one in the maxillary anterior region was very high. This was fully explained to the patient during the doctor–patient conference, so that treatment could be performed on the basis of informed consent.

Once the maxillary right and left permanent central incisors were aligned, a large "black triangle" did appear. The contact area was reproximated using hand strips and rotary instrumentation to both lengthen it incisoapically and broaden it faciolingually. Elastomeric thread was then used to close the diastema and "pinch" the interdental papilla incisally. This technique greatly reduced the size of the "black triangle" but did not fully eliminate it. This specific dentofacial trait had poor therapeutic modifiability, which was discussed with the patient prior to instituting therapy.

Table 6.28 Patient Data

Age	24 Years, 4 months
Chief complaint	"Appearance of front teeth"
Medical history	Noncontributory
Dental history	Oral hygiene within normal limits
	Low caries rate
	Dental visits at 6-month intervals
	Orthodontic treatment for 2 years as an adolescent (four premolar extraction)
	Third molar removal
	Temporomandibular joint dysfunction, wears a mandibular anterior repositioning appliance (MARA)

Table 6.29 Orthognal Analysis

Dentofacial appearance	Unattractive incisor display (tooth No. 9)
Alignment	Thin/scalloped periodontal biotype
	Maxillary left permanent central incisor (tooth No. 9) labioverted and 1 mm longer than the right permanent central incisor (tooth No. 8)
	Mild mandibular rotations "black triangles" in the mandibular anterior interdental spaces
Transverse	No deviation
Sagittal	Class II molar left side
Vertical	Anterior deep bite

Table 6.30 Enhancement Outcome

Primary Characteristic	Specific Variation	Enhancement
Dentofacial appearance	Unattractive anterior tooth display (tooth No. 9)	Tooth movement improved the position of tooth No. 9
Alignment	Tooth No. 9 labioverted and extruded	Aligned tooth No. 9
	Thin/scalloped periodontal biotype	Reproximation of the contact between tooth No. 8 and tooth No. 9 improved the maxillary anterior "black triangle" but did not eliminate it

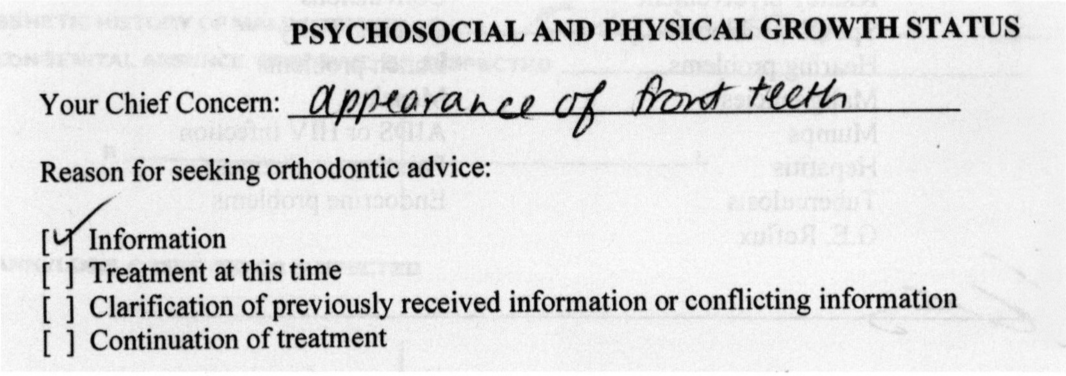

PSYCHOSOCIAL AND PHYSICAL GROWTH STATUS

Your Chief Concern: *appearance of front teeth*

Reason for seeking orthodontic advice:

[✓] Information
[ ] Treatment at this time
[ ] Clarification of previously received information or conflicting information
[ ] Continuation of treatment

Figure 6.50 The patient's chief concern and reason for seeking orthodontic advice.

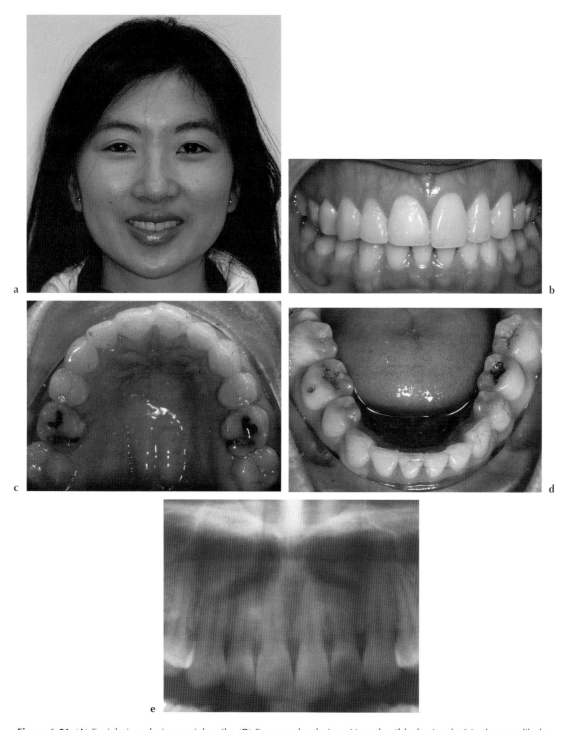

Figure 6.51 (**A**) Facial view during social smile. (**B**) Front occlusal view. Note the "black triangles" in the mandibular anterior interdental spaces. (**C**) Maxillary occlusal view. (**D**) Mandibular occlusal view. (**E**) Cropped panoramic radiograph pretreatment. In healthy oral cavities, the gingival papillae fill the space between the teeth 100% of the time when the distance from the contact point of the adjacent teeth to the interproximal crest of the bone is 5 mm or less. When the distance is 6 mm, the papillae do not fill the space completely in approximately 50% of patients, and when it is 7 mm or more, it does not fill the space in 75% of patients (Tarnow et al. 1992). In this patient, the distance from the contact point (teeth No. 8 and No. 9) to the interproximal crest of bone exceeds 6 mm.

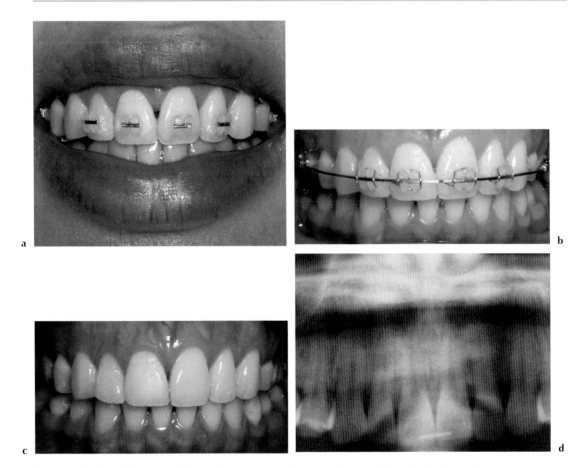

Figure 6.52 (**A**) A "black triangle" developed after leveling teeth No. 8 and No. 9. (**B**) The teeth were reproximated and the resultant diastema closed. (**C**) Occlusal view at debond. (**D**) Cropped post-treatment panoramic radiograph.

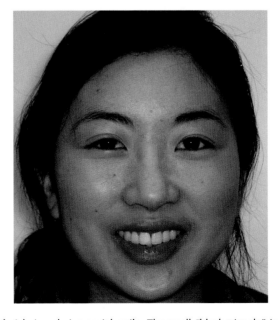

Figure 6.53 Post-treatment facial view during social smile. The small "black triangle" is visible between teeth No. 8 and No. 9.

REFERENCES

Ackerman, J.L., Proffit, W.R. 1997. Soft tissue limitations in orthodontics: Treatment planning guidelines. *Angle Orthod* 67:327–336.

Rosen, H.M. 1992. Facial skeletal expansion: Treatment strategies and rationale. *Plast Reconstr Surg* 89:798–808.

Swick, M.D., Richter, A. 2003. A comparative study of two intraoral laser techniques for soft tissue laser surgery. *Proc SPIE* 4950:11–17.

Afterword

It is the hope of this Author that the readers of this volume gained a greater appreciation for the theory and practice of enhancement orthodontics. Several warmly held concepts in dentistry, and in particular orthodontics, have been challenged in this work. Conspicuously absent from this text are the terms *malocclusion*, *esthetics*, and *cephalometrics*. These concepts have confused and confounded, rather than defined and clarified, the nature of orthodontics. The term *malocclusion* has been replaced with variation in dentofacial traits because orthodontic conditions should be viewed on a continuum rather than described on an either/or basis relative only to "ideal" occlusion. The term dentofacial appearance has been substituted for *esthetics* because of clearer meaning. Lastly, *cephalometrics* was excluded from this volume because it is the practice of pseudo-scientific measurement based on mean values that do not have significant import when applied to the individual.

Although the perspective on orthodontics advocated in this book may seem radical to the casual reader, a glimpse into orthodontic history reveals that it is hardly a new idea.

"Theoretically, dentistry is a science and an art. Practically, to a very great extent, it has been empiricism in place of science, and bungling mechanism in place of art."
Norman W. Kingsley, *A Treatise on Oral Deformities as a Branch of Mechanical Surgery* (1880)

"To no one does the study of the human face, in its various forms and aspects, recommend itself with more force than to the dental practitioner; for, called upon as he is, not only to relieve suffering humanity from the greatest pain to which flesh is heir, but also to repair the ravages of decay, either in efforts directed toward the preservation of the natural organs, or, when these are lost, to supply artificial substitutes, if he is not as quick to perceive and as able to retain in his memory the nice shades of expression of the same face, and the characteristic points of resemblance or difference between various individuals, as the sculptor or painter, he will fail in many essential particulars to meet all the just and proper demands upon him."
Norman W. Kingsley, *A Treatise on Oral Deformities as a Branch of Mechanical Surgery* (1880)

"The success of orthodontia as a science and an art now lies in the retainer."
Norman W. Kingsley, December 3rd, 1908, in a letter to the Alumni Society of the Angle School of Orthodontia

Index